How to Eat
(and Still Lose Weight)

A Science-Backed Guide to Nutrition
and Health

DR ANDREW JENKINSON

PENGUIN LIFE

AN IMPRINT OF

PENGUIN BOOKS

For Dad, my Superhero

PENGUIN LIFE

UK | USA | Canada | Ireland | Australia
India | New Zealand | South Africa

Penguin Life is part of the Penguin Random House group of companies
whose addresses can be found at global.penguinrandomhouse.com

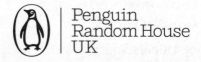

Penguin
Random House
UK

First published 2024
001

Copyright © Andrew Jenkinson, 2024
Illustrations copyright © Malcolm Willett @ The Rubicon

The moral right of the copyright holders has been asserted

This book is based on my own experience as a consultant surgeon with
a special interest in advanced laparoscopic, or keyhole, surgery. In order to protect
the privacy and confidence of patients, I have, of course, not used any real names
and I have changed all physical descriptions and other features to ensure that
no one is identifiable. I have, in some cases, also changed genders and
racial origins. This is because this is not a book about the individuals I have
described, but about what we can learn from them

Set in 12/14.75pt Dante MT Std
Typeset by Jouve (UK), Milton Keynes
Printed and bound in Great Britain by Clays Ltd, Elcograf S.p.A.

The authorized representative in the EEA is Penguin Random House Ireland,
Morrison Chambers, 32 Nassau Street, Dublin D02 YH68

A CIP catalogue record for this book is available from the British Library

ISBN: 978-0-241-62798-3

www.greenpenguin.co.uk

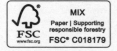

Contents

Contents

Prologue

The New Fuel

Imagine that a New Fuel has been developed that can be used instead of petrol in your car. The New Fuel is much cheaper than petrol and seems to work just as well. The day-to-day performance of your car appears unaffected. The only issue is that the New Fuel doesn't last for as long as petrol, but despite the need to refuel more frequently it is still much more cost-effective per mile. The New Fuel immediately becomes popular.

Because the New Fuel is so cheap, the producers are able to offer an additional reward to buyers. A small gift that makes the car owner happy is provided at the pump every time they fill up. Clever advertising by the New Fuel companies also suggests other benefits of using it. The advertising works, and New Fuel users feel good when they fill up their cars.

As well as giving you a satisfying feeling when you refuel, the advertising campaigns start to make it feel normal to fill up more frequently. Billboards and TV ads appear of happy, beautiful people going to New Fuel stations daily, and feeling great when they do this, changing the behaviour of car drivers. It is no longer considered normal to fill up with petrol every week or so; instead the required daily refill of the cheap New Fuel becomes normal behaviour. To make things easier, New Fuel stations become available every few miles . . . and your gas tank can be filled up in a matter of seconds through modern high-pressure pumps.

Some companies offer to adapt your car so that it can hold much more of the New Fuel. Larger gas tanks are added to the outsides of cars, bulking up the doors and trunks. Although this makes driving more hazardous and slow, it catches on. Within a few years, a third of the cars on the road have been adapted so that they dwarf standard cars.

And so a whole industry around the New Fuel emerges, encouraging its use, reassuring us that it is safe, changing our refuelling behaviour and adapting our cars to have massive fuel tanks.

But if you looked under the bonnet of your car and really examined its inner workings, you would realize that it was never really designed to run on the New Fuel. You would see that the New Fuel damages the engine, meaning it is less powerful (and needs even more New Fuel to perform). The fuel seeps out of the tanks into the body of the car, accelerating corrosion and rust, and ageing the car prematurely. It interferes with the electronics, meaning the massive storage tanks always appear nearly empty on the fuel gauge. After a few years of use, the engine splutters and behaves erratically. The massive new fuel tanks make the car unstable and unsafe to drive. It dies early.

The New Foods

Just like cars, humans need fuel to survive and move. Fuel in the form of food. Over the last few decades, new types of human foods have emerged. Processed foods – made up primarily of sugar, refined carbohydrates (such as wheat), vegetable oils, and artificial flavourings and colourings – now dominate the nutritional options available to us. These foods are mass-produced in factories, marketed aggressively and packaged colourfully. They are addictive to humans and highly profitable for the food industry. They appear, over the short term, to be safe – our bodies can easily run on them. And just like in the New Fuel story above, these New Foods are cheap, they make us feel good, and we are encouraged by advertising to eat them more frequently. But just like in the car analogy, the New Foods cause major dysfunction in how our bodies work.

This book will lift the lid on our own human bonnet, explaining how the tasty, addictive New Foods around us disrupt our bodies and our minds. We'll learn how we are not designed to run on them, and how they cause our bodies to misfire and our brains to miscalculate. They make us feel unnaturally good but force many of us to need extra fuel stores (in the form of fat); and for others they cause oxidative corrosion and modern Western diseases . . . In other words, they make us die early.

Once you understand this, you will want to eat – in fact you will crave – the foods we are designed to run on. You will not want to consume the New Foods. The mental shift in your understanding of how your body uses fuel means that minimal willpower will be needed to change. You will finally understand how your own body – your own personal engine – works.

In this book I'll show you how to choose healthier foods and offer tips and techniques for incorporating them into your diet, helping you to lose weight in the process, if that is your goal. With these powerful insights in hand, your body will revert to the wonderful machine it was made to be . . .

Introduction

'If you know the enemy and know yourself, you need not fear the result of a hundred battles. If you know yourself but not the enemy, for every victory gained you will also suffer a defeat. If you know neither the enemy nor yourself, you will succumb in every battle.'

Sun Tzu, *The Art of War*

Ain Al Khaleej Hospital, Al Ain, UAE, January 2022

We were basking in the evening sun, sitting together on a bench outside the main entrance, taking a break from a long clinic. The hospital had a curious space-age design. It looked like a giant cylindrical UFO that had just landed. Around it were immaculate lawns that abutted neatly painted zebra kerbstones. A vividly colourful flower-bedded roundabout stood next to the main entrance, welcoming incoming 4x4s and luxury cars. In and out of the sliding doors wandered Emirati men, clad head to toe in white robes, and their wives, fully covered in black burqas.

Since early morning we had been visited by patient after patient after patient – a long line of people who sensed they had lost control of their weight and were becoming sicker and sadder because of it. With the help of Samer, my Jordanian friend and Arabic translator, we had explained, again and again, the most effective ways to lose weight. Either by changing diet, injection treatment or weight-loss surgery (like gastric bypass).

Samer took a sip of his strong Turkish coffee and said something astonishing to me. 'Do you know, Dr Andrew, that I too used to suffer with obesity. I weighed 125kg [around 20 stone].' He then proceeded to describe to me exactly how he was able to turn his situation around. How, by understanding how his body, and just as importantly, how his mind worked, he had been able to devise a way to sustain his weight loss for the past ten years.

Samer now weighed 70kg (11 stone) and looked great – tanned, happy and healthy. Every day he dressed in a different dapper suit that showed off his tall, slim frame. His inquisitive outlook on life and his attitude towards his journey through extreme weight gain and then weight loss was compelling. The basis of his success was very similar to the advice I give patients, outlined in my first book, *Why We Eat (Too Much): The New Science of Appetite*. But he had never read the book; instead he had worked out how to reset his weight through years of trying. He achieved the same weight loss that would be expected after bariatric surgery, the operations we had been describing to our Emirati patients all day . . . but he had never undergone this surgery.

Sensing my enthusiasm for his story, Samer charted his weight-gain journey in more detail. When he was younger he had lived in Jordan, in a time before much junk food was available. In his early twenties he would work during the day, then play football in the streets in the evening, before coming home at dusk to fill himself up with tasty grilled meats and fish, rice and flatbread, yogurt and tabbouleh, finishing off with coffee and fresh fruit. At sunrise he would wake up to strong Arabic tea and dates.

Aged twenty-six, he relocated to the United Arab Emirates, taking a job as a chief operating theatre technician in a pristine new hospital. His whole lifestyle changed. The UAE is hot like a furnace in the summer, and so people tend to stay in their air-conditioned apartments. For Samer there was no football, and no home-prepared food to come back to in the evening. At first he loved the new foods available to him – fast foods that tasted so good, sweet snacks that made him feel great and deflected his loneliness. He got into the habit of ordering fast-food deliveries in the evening. And then the Netflix revolution came about and he spent most evenings binge-watching his latest favourite TV show while mindlessly eating snacks. His weight went from 80kg, to 90, to 100, to 115, before settling at 125kg.

Over the next ten years, he dieted. He tried all the latest fad diets, starved himself, and exercised. His weight yo-yoed up and down by 10–12kg during this time, but the excess pounds always came back. As Samer said of one particular diet he'd tried, 'Keto was like breathing in and out of a balloon; the weight goes down and up, down and up.'

One morning he was listening to a local Arabic radio station and they were discussing the health benefits of taking a drink of hot water with fresh lemon juice on waking, and not eating for a full hour afterwards. His interest was piqued, as his colleague at work had told him just that week that this remedy had helped kick start significant weight loss by helping 'melt away' the fat. He tried it and some weight came off.* He had finally started to nourish himself and become aware of his body.

Inspired by this small victory, Samer decided to address his late-night snack habit. But it proved difficult to just give up this ingrained behaviour, so instead of cutting out his evening snack, he switched from sweets and crisps to preparing a board of sliced carrots, cucumbers and finely chopped raw cabbage

---

* It would have had great antioxidant effects and also increased his period of fasting, making him feel better in himself and stimulating some weight loss.

with a sprinkle of salt. After two months of doing this he noticed further weight loss. Eventually he was able to stop snacking in the evening entirely and decided to get early nights to give his body time to rest and repair itself. Some further weight loss followed, but then he hit a plateau of 105kg.

His next move was the most difficult. He correctly reasoned that sugar was not good for his metabolism and decided to avoid it completely. 'Losing weight is like a war,' he told me. 'You will win it with strategy and being clever and understanding the body.' He smiled. 'When I gave up sugar my friends laughed at me and tempted me with treats – I wanted to cry, I wanted to hit my head against a wall, but after forty days the addiction was gone. It became easy. If you stop sugar for forty days you will never want it again. But it takes a strong mind to do this.'

Samer's weight hit 90kg but again plateaued. He realized that exercise was not shifting his weight. 'Two hours on the treadmill is the same as one Coca-Cola. It's not for weight loss but is good to keep the muscles tight.'

One of the rules that he came to like was his theory that 'if it tastes too good it will probably harm the body, but if it tastes natural it is good for you'. He became mindful of the tastes of different foods and began to crave natural foods and dislike processed food. 'If a fast-food burger was in front of me and it was the last thing on earth to eat, I would leave it.' He gave up white rice, sensing that it was too heavy, and exchanged it for bulgur wheat which he found 'lighter on the stomach'. He started to consume just two meals per day of fresh foods, and would not eat for the two hours before bed. 'Each meal you should not eat so much that you want to sleep,' he said.

Even though he was aware that vigorous exercise was not a long-term weight-loss solution, he was aware of the benefits of moderate exercise, which he believed 'wakes up the body and is good for the metabolism, even a walk'. He said you should try to 'reach an addiction that is opposite to bad food – not just eating good food but craving restful sleep and savouring exercise'.

His weight came down to 80kg and stayed like this for several months. Then, over a matter of weeks, without any further changes to his diet, he lost more weight as his body finally adapted to his new lifestyle, settling at 70kg. Over the past ten years he had successfully maintained a healthy weight of between 70 and 75kg.

What intrigued me most was that the successful changes that he had made in his lifestyle and diet only came about after a shift in his mentality – the way he thought about food and his health. After years of trial and error, years of failed diets, Samer had come to understand that the most important battle to win was the one in the mind. His weight-loss success was not based on an unusually iron willpower (although he had needed some willpower initially to give up sugar); it was based on a change in his outlook and understanding of food. He did not feel as if he was giving anything up; he felt no loss for the foods he had eaten before. He craved healthy food now, and was turned off by the taste and the feeling that unhealthy foods gave him. 'You need to become addicted to healthy foods, just like you were addicted before to junk food. Your mind and your body will thank you for it.'

Samer continued with gems of dietary advice every time we met. It seemed he had reached a new way of living; he had changed as a person and his body had changed with him. At first it had taken some self-discipline, but eventually it became easy for him. 'Weight loss is like learning to play the guitar,' he said. 'The more you practise, the better you will get at it. You should not be disheartened when things don't always go to plan.'

My discussions with Samer inspired me to write this book.

Once you clearly understand how the toxic food environment surrounding you affects your body and your mind, it becomes much easier to lose weight *and* keep that weight off for good. It's easier to sustain weight loss if you truly understand how your mind and your body react to unhealthy foods. How these addictive foods can influence your metabolism, your appetite, your behaviour and your habits. How these habits can be hard to break. In *How to Eat*, alongside a new understanding of how we function (or malfunction) in our current environment, I will provide a tactical rulebook to follow that clearly outlines how to make healthy changes to your lifestyle that will stick.

Many people who read my last book, *Why We Eat (Too Much)*, were full of praise for how it changed their lives; it was a tool to help them adjust their weight to a healthier level over the long term. I received hundreds of messages from people who were able to implement the book's ideas in their daily lives and to lose a considerable amount of weight (and keep it off). 'Pretty mind blowing', 'should be on medical students' syllabus' and 'the Rosetta Stone of modern human health!' were just some of the reviews posted on Amazon. However, other people tried their best to follow the guidance but found themselves dragged back to old behaviours. *Why We Eat* described the relationship between our food and our bodies, but not how our brains work to constantly seek the easy, familiar, pleasurable path, often to the detriment of our health. *How to Eat* will unpack the new, vitally important science of the brain and the body, showing you how to harness your body and reprogramme your mind to lose weight for good.

Since *Why We Eat* was published, scientists have made great strides in understanding how the brain makes decisions, including how reward pathways are etched permanently into our brains and how these pathways lead to habitual and mindless behaviours. We have also learned how behaviours are triggered by cues or reminders that if we take such an action we will get a reward, generating a pleasant feeling in us. An example of this, outside of the food-health area, is our growing use of smartphones. These devices are designed to trigger a little feeling of pleasure (a dopamine hit) whenever a nice message or a funny video comes up. Hence many (probably most) people are constantly checking their phones to see if that message or video is there. I am increasingly amazed that if you look at a group of people in a public place, most of them will be gazing at their phones, looking for that pleasure trigger. Sometimes I too find myself gazing at the phone screen, almost like a zombie, in my habit loop. In this book, we will examine how processed foods can trigger those same pleasure-centres, and how they can cause unhealthy habits to form. We will learn how our habit loops are exploited by the food industry for its profit, with unfortunate consequences for our health and wellbeing.

How to Eat (and Still Lose Weight) will explore and explain how our decision-making works, how unhealthy habitual behaviours form, and more importantly how to replace them with healthier behaviours. We will delve into addictions – how to recognize them and how to overcome them. One of the important areas in this field is the trigger – the cue or reminder – in our environment that makes our brain crave a certain reward and follow a certain action. We will examine how food companies are not only experts in making foods that act like drugs, giving us a temporary high, but also able to create the trigger (or trap) in the first place, through well-placed adverts and clever marketing. By understanding these traps for what they are, and why they are placed – as well as the health consequences of falling into them – we will be much better prepared to cope with the constant bombardment of temptation. This knowledge will promote a new outlook and understanding – a form of identity change that will cause a natural desire for a healthier eating pattern. It will give you the tools to create that aversion to modern foods that my friend Samer described, so that no willpower is needed to change.

The book also covers *how* to change once you have this knowledge: how to change unhealthy habits, how to cope with cravings, and how to relax without resorting to food or drugs. It will make clear what foods to try to avoid and what foods to savour. Hopefully, by this time, your understanding of food will make this easy.

A common theme of the feedback from my first book was that it was not prescriptive enough. Many readers wanted more specific examples of meals and meal plans. In the final chapter, Global Kitchen, chefs have helped me to identify some wonderfully nutritious breakfast, lunch and dinner ideas from around the world to provide a great new variety of choices for you.

Finally, I would like to emphasize that this is not purely a book about weight. We know modern foods not only cause obesity (in about a quarter of the population), they are also the cause of many diseases not commonly seen in the areas of the world that have maintained their traditional food culture. Many autoimmune diseases, inflammatory conditions and allergies are directly caused by our modern food environment. By changing the way you eat and live, you will be protecting yourself against these conditions.

As Sun Tzu wrote in *The Art of War*, if you know your enemy and yourself, you need not fear the result of a hundred battles. Once you have read this book, you will know how your body and your mind work, and you will understand exactly how modern food and the modern food environment affect you. You should not fear, or doubt, the outcome.

PART I

Body

How We Adjust to Modern Food

CHAPTER I

Diet School

Understanding Weight Control

*Operating Theatre 10, University College London
Hospital, January 2023*

Mr Johnson weighed around 150kg (23½ stone). He had
informed me that he had always been on the big side but just
could not lose weight when he carried out the instructions of
the numerous dieticians, nutritionists, fitness instructors and
life coaches he had seen in the past. He had recently developed
diabetes and had decided to seek a referral to my bariatric
surgery unit at University College London Hospital. His
semi-naked body was now being carefully prepared for that
surgery.

Every muscle in his body had been paralysed by an injection
of curare, the same ancient plant poison used by Amazonian
hunters in their blow darts. Because of his paralysis, he couldn't
breathe now and so was connected to the breathing machine
via a throat tube, its bellows providing a reassuring sound to
my friend Wint, our anaesthetist. She had administered a form
of hypnotic (the same compound found in so-called date rape
drugs) so that all memory of this event would be erased. She
had topped him up with a hefty shot of morphine in anticipation of the pain to come.

He was lying flat on the operating table with his arms out-stretched and legs apart, almost as if mid-star jump. I was reminded of Leonardo da Vinci's famous *Vitruvian Man* sketch, but this time with a very large modern-day individual. As the theatre staff secured the patient's arms and legs to the table extensions with soft crêpe bandages, I stood between his legs and took the operating-table remote control, pressing the 'Reverse Trendelenburg' button. The table whirred and Mr Johnson was elevated to a 45-degree angle, his body robotically rotating to face towards me. A large TV monitor attached to a hinged metal arm was swung down to a comfortable viewing position just below my eyeline and about a metre away from me.

Lise, our senior scrub nurse, wheeled in a trolley laden with surgical blades, clips, tubes and wires, to rest next to Mr Johnson's body, and she proceeded to apply bright orange skin-disinfectant to his rotund abdomen. The surgical lights came on, brightly illuminating the whole area, and green sterile drapes were positioned around Mr Johnson's body and legs so that the only skin visible was the orange luminescent square of his abdomen. It was time for theatre, time to perform, to con-centrate and operate. I went to the scrub sink to get clean.

Gowned, gloved and masked, everything was set. I stood between Mr Johnson's legs, holding a razor-sharp surgical blade next to his abdominal skin. 'Is it OK to start, Wint?' I asked. At her nod, the gleaming blade sliced a 12mm (half-inch) cut through his skin and he bled healthy bright red blood. 'Trocar, please.' Lise handed me a see-through plastic tube with a pointed end, almost like a blunt pencil point. I placed a thin surgical telescope (the instrument relaying the images of the surgery, via a digital camera, to the TV monitor) into the plastic tube and aimed the pencil point through the bleeding cut I had made in Mr Johnson's abdomen. I looked at the TV monitor and could see that we were at the level of the yellow fat under his skin. At this stage I proceeded to carefully stab Mr Johnson all the way through his abdominal wall with the pencil-like implement, putting my weight into it, twisting and forcing its sharp point deep into him. If he hadn't signed the consent form agreeing for me to do this to him, it would have been a criminal assault. But as it was, the stabbing was agreed, and controlled, and each layer of his abdominal wall – fat–fascia–muscle–fat – was visible to me on the screen as the trocar slipped safely into his abdomen.

The procedure I was about to perform would be life-changing for Mr Johnson. A year from this day, after I surgically removed most of his stomach, he would weigh around 90kg (just over 14 stone), his diabetes would have disappeared, he would not feel hungry or crave bad food, and his self-esteem and quality of life would be immeasurably improved.

I made four more small cuts into his skin and stabbed four more pencil-point trocars through his abdominal wall. Through one of the trocars, a tube pumping carbon dioxide gas into the abdomen was placed. As the gas entered Mr Johnson's abdominal cavity, his abdomen ballooned on the outside to resemble a full-term pregnancy, and on the inside the gas created the space to vividly see his organs and to perform the operation. Then the surgical lights were turned off and the operating theatre became like a dark movie theatre; the crisp digital HD images of Mr Johnson's insides gleamed on TV monitors throughout the room, and a hush descended, the only sound the beep-beep-beep of the heart monitor.

We had an audience today – two young medical students who had been watching the whole process since Mr Johnson was wheeled into theatre. It was half a lifetime since I had been in their position, but I knew they were excited and scared at the same time. I wanted to make sure they remembered and learned from their experience. I started by pointing the camera at Mr Johnson's purple and engorged liver. 'Twenty per cent of obese people have this type of liver. It's due to too much fat and sugar storage and can cause inflammation, and liver cirrhosis in the future.' I swung the camera to point out the omentum – the glistening and inflamed yellow fat hanging like an apron from the large bowel – as well as the dusky spleen throbbing away like a potential vascular explosion, and his vast pink stomach.

'This operation is called a sleeve gastrectomy,' I told the students. 'Basically, we are going to remove around two-thirds to three-quarters of his stomach.' They were staring at the TV monitor as I indicated the sizeable part of the stomach that was going to be removed. 'The stomach will be reduced in capacity from the size of a Galia melon to the size of a banana,* going from a 2-litre capacity to around 200 to 300cc . . . but the question I want to ask you is why is this man having this surgery in the first place? Why can't he just go on a diet and move more?'

'Maybe he tried but lacked the willpower to lose weight on a diet,' one replied. 'Could it be that he has a food addiction?' the other answered.

---

* Doctors often describe the size of a lump, cyst or organ by comparing it to the size of a fruit – grape, plum, tangerine, orange and melon being common examples. Very occasionally a sporty surgeon will use sports balls as a comparison; golf ball, tennis ball, etc. 'His hernia is the size of a . . . tangerine / tennis ball / grapefruit / rugby ball [delete as appropriate].'

Leptin – The Fat Hormone

'Haven't they taught you anything about *leptin* in medical school yet?' I enquired. After a long pause, one of the students replied, 'Oh yes, we had a lecture which mentioned it. I think it comes from fat cells and influences appetite, but that's all we were told.' I silently shook my head – still the medical schools were not explaining obesity to their students.

I started to dissect the outer edge of Mr Johnson's stomach away from its fat and blood vessels using a harmonic coagulator, an instrument whose pincers rub the tissues grasped between them at 55,000 times per second, causing heat, thermal injury and good coagulation, stopping any blood vessels in its jaws from bleeding. As the tissues were cleanly cut, smoke from the vaporizing fat started to cloud the view, so I opened the smoke-extractor valve.

'Well, leptin is the *master controller* of our weight, and when it stops working properly people lose control of their weight no matter what they try and do about it. Leptin is a hormone that comes from fat, and the more fat someone has, the higher the leptin level in the blood.' I grasped Mr Johnson's abdominal belly fat between my finger and thumb to demonstrate. 'This man has a lot of fat and so will have a lot of leptin in his system. But leptin is the hormone that is supposed to stop people getting too fat, or too thin. The amount of leptin in the blood acts as a signal to the part of the brain that controls our weight called the *hypothalamus*. The hypothalamus controls how hungry or full we feel. You know that feeling after you've finished a large meal? The feeling of fullness you still feel three hours after you have finished eating, even when the stomach is empty? That full feeling comes from your hypothalamus. What about that feeling when you have been so busy that you didn't eat all day, and then in the evening you are so hungry, you will eat anything? That feeling, that signal to act and to eat, comes from our hypothalamus. Hormones are very good at reminding us what to do.

'So, when things are working normally, your hypothalamus will be able to sense if you have put some weight on. It will sense the increase in the leptin level in the blood and will respond by increasing feelings of fullness, and decrease your appetite. The response is that you naturally eat less and you seamlessly lose the weight that you had gained, until your leptin level returns to normal. Leptin is just the signal to your brain telling it how much fat you have stored – how much energy is available in the future. It acts like the fuel gauge on your car dashboard. When the gauge is full, you have no interest in filling up, but once the gauge dips towards empty you will be looking to fill the tank back up.'

The Broken Gas Tank Meter – Leptin Resistance

'So, if leptin is so good at supressing appetite and controlling your weight, what has happened to this signal in Mr Johnson? His leptin level would be very high if we measured it.' I looked

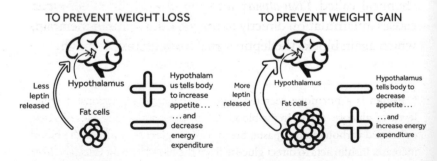

Figure 1: Leptin ensures normal weight control

up from the stomach dissection, I had nearly got to the top of the stomach and was negotiating the tricky short gastric blood vessels connecting it to the spleen. The students seemed to be stumped by this question . . . then one suggested that the leptin signal might somehow be being blocked.

'Yes! You are getting there. Mr Johnson has a condition called *leptin resistance*. He has lots of leptin in his blood but it is not being seen by his brain. It's being hidden. And the culprit is the hormone *insulin*.* Leptin and insulin have a common signalling pathway within the hypothalamus. If insulin levels are high, then the insulin will block the receptor on the hypothalamus that leptin is supposed to activate. Mr Johnson has a typical Western diet that includes lots of sugar and refined carbohydrates, which are sugar precursors. In addition, he will be much more likely to snack between meals. Lots of sugar and snacking leads to lots of insulin being produced, and that insulin blocks the leptin signal from getting through.'

'That's just the first way that the leptin signal is blocked.' I pointed to the TV monitor, and focused in on the gleaming fat hanging off Mr Johnson's stomach. 'You see this fat looks abnormal – it's too moist, it's inflamed, and the inflammation is caused by his obesity. All this fatty inflammation sends a chemical called *TNF-alpha*† into the blood. The TNF-alpha causes inflammation directly to the hypothalamus in the brain, which again blocks the leptin signal from getting through.'

---

* Insulin is a hormone secreted from the pancreas in response to high levels of glucose (sugar) in the blood. After a meal containing a lot of sugar or refined carbohydrates (pasta, bread, cakes), glucose levels in the blood increase. Insulin acts to direct glucose from the blood into fat cells (and liver and muscle), to store this energy for future use.
† Tumour necrosis factor alpha.

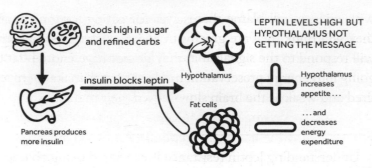

Figure 2: Uncontrolled weight gain from sugars

I had finished the surgical dissection; the stomach was now mobilized enough for its division to begin.

Leptin Resistance = The Disease Obesity

'So, Mr Johnson has the condition that we call leptin resistance, and what I would call the *disease obesity*. He has far too much fat on board, and therefore has produced high levels of leptin. But due to the nature of his diet, that high leptin signal is being blocked by insulin. He has stored more and more fat, and this has led to inflammation of the fat and inflammation of the hypothalamus, blocking the leptin signal even more. His hypothalamus cannot see the leptin, and therefore cannot sense that he is storing too much fat. In fact, the opposite is true – his brain is getting the signal that there is *not enough* leptin. It is getting signals that he does *not* have enough fat storage.

'Most people suffering with obesity are getting signals to eat more. Their appetite is high all the time. It's embarrassing for them to eat too much in public, so quite often they will binge-eat in private. And because doctors and society in general don't understand the chemical pathways that lead to obesity, people with obesity will blame themselves for eating too much, and they will think they are greedy. In addition, the hypothalamus will respond to the signals that they do not have enough fat by going into energy preservation mode. This will make them feel tired and weak as the brain slows down their metabolism.'

> Understanding leptin resistance is crucial to being able to control your weight. Sustained weight loss is not about calorie counting (we know low-calorie diets don't work long-term), it's about altering the food that you eat so that your normal system of weight regulation is restored. If you can do this, your weight will naturally reset to a healthier level without any unpleasant feelings of hunger or of missing out.

I explained that leptin acts like the fuel meter signal in your car. Imagine driving along the motorway and you notice the fuel meter flashing empty. You immediately start looking for a gas station (in leptin resistance you would feel hungry), and you might be so worried that you will break down before you can fill up that you start driving slower to preserve fuel (in leptin resistance you would feel tired). When you get to the petrol pump and start to fill up, you realize that the tank is already full and the problem is that your fuel meter is faulty. But in leptin resistance this does not happen; there is no automatic shut-off to over-refuelling as there is at the gas station. The low leptin signal is very real, and despite having plenty of energy reserves in the form of fat you continue to refuel, eating more and more but never seeming to be able to satisfy that hunger . . . leading to further uncontrolled weight gain.

Leptin

Leptin is the hormone that keeps control of your weight by informing your brain how much energy you are storing. The leptin signal is blocked by too much insulin in the blood. If you consume a diet that increases insulin, then your body will misread the leptin signal as low and you will take in too many calories and gain weight. Insulin is increased by consuming too much sugar, too many foods containing refined carbohydrates (such as wheat) and too much vegetable oil. These foods do not cause weight gain because they contain too many calories. They lead to weight gain because of the confusion they cause to your normal weight-control signalling.

'Mr Johnson weighs over 23 stone, has an unhealthy appetite and is tired all the time,' I said to the students. 'Our conventional and too simplified understanding of obesity would point to his supposed greed and laziness as being character flaws *causing* his obesity. But in actual fact his exposure to the Western diet and snacking culture has disrupted the normal control his body would have to stop him storing too much fat. The condition he has developed due to the type of food he is exposed to – leptin resistance, or what I would call the disease obesity – causes the *symptoms* of voracious hunger and tiredness. As a result, too much energy is taken in and too little energy is used, *leading* to uncontrolled weight gain. This is the problem with obesity – people blame greed and laziness for causing it but it is a condition that *causes* this behaviour. These are its symptoms, not its cause. Just like the symptoms of a cold might be a cough and a fever.'

It was time to staple Mr Johnson's stomach. I asked Wint to push a large hosepipe-sized tube through his mouth, down his oesophagus (gullet) and into his stomach. As the tube passed through the length of his stomach, I straightened it using my surgical graspers. I would be using this tube to guide my staple position and calibrate the size of the new stomach.

'Stapler, please.' Lise placed the stapler's handle directly into my outstretched hand as I kept my eyes on the image of the stomach on the TV monitor in front of me. As I passed the long narrow staple machine through one of the trocar tubes and into Mr Johnson's abdomen, I saw it appear on the screen. I opened the crocodile-like jaws of the stapler and carefully positioned it at the lower end of the stomach, noticing that it was sitting just the right distance from the calibration tube. The jaws closed and I pulled the automatic trigger of the battery-powered staple gun; the staples and knife whirred, simultaneously cutting through the stomach and sealing it with small rows of titanium staples. Several more staples were neatly fired until the top of the stomach, close to the oesophagus had been reached. The last of the staple firings separated the stomach into two – the small tube-like new stomach that would remain, and the bulk of the old stomach that was to be removed. Without its blood supply, this part was already turning a dusky blue due to lack of oxygen.

The students were concentrating intently on the screen while listening to my explanation of leptin resistance as a cause of Mr Johnson's current predicament. 'But if he was somehow *forced* to eat less and *forced* to exercise, he would lose weight, wouldn't he?' one of them asked.

'Yes, of course he would,' I said. 'But all the time that he is losing weight, his body would be fighting weight loss. There is an appetite hormone called *ghrelin* that comes from this part of the stomach' – I pointed to the top part of the stomach that I had just detached – 'and this hormone would increase significantly and signal to the hypothalamus to cause a voracious appetite and food-seeking behaviour. It is basically directing the person's actions to make him eat more and stop any more weight loss, and these signals are very powerful and it's difficult to resist them. This is why most people who lose weight on a diet can't continue it for very long. If Mr Johnson were locked up and he had no choice because he couldn't access food, then he would suffer with these feelings and continue losing weight. His metabolism would collapse, meaning he would feel very tired and weak as his body did all it could to preserve as much energy as possible. As soon as he was released into his normal food environment, he would eat ravenously in response to his hunger signals, until he had regained all the weight he had lost. This is what happens to most people when they describe dieting.'

It was now time to test whether the staples that we had used to remove most of the stomach were working. The remaining stomach resembled a narrow cylinder,* and I asked Wint to flush a blue-coloured liquid through the tube and into the new stomach to see if it was leaking from anywhere. It seemed intact, there was no leakage.

I continued: 'The problem with Mr Johnson and all people who suffer with obesity is that the weight that they are is what their brain thinks is a healthy weight. This is called their *weight set-point*.'

---

* The operation is called a sleeve gastrectomy because the stomach, after it has been cut, resembles a sleeve.

Your Own Weight Setting

'Every person has their own individual weight set-point,' I told the students. *'This is the weight that your brain wants you to be.* If you are lucky, your weight set-point is in the normal range. If you overindulge and put weight on, your brain will stop you eating too much – by signalling satiety – and if you have lost weight through sickness your brain ensures weight regain by increasing your appetite. By doing this, your brain ensures that you will remain a healthy weight for years and years without having to think too much about calories. Your brain automatically calculates whether it wants energy in your body or whether it wants you to stop eating and expend energy instead – in just the same way your brain will tell you how much to drink by adjusting your thirst according to whether you are dehydrated or not.'

I explained that the problem comes if your weight set-point is in the overweight or obese category.* 'If this happens, then every effort to force your weight down by simple calorie restriction and exercise will ultimately fail. This is because your brain will fight against the weight loss of dieting, as it wants to keep your weight at its set-point because it thinks this is safer for you.'

---

* Doctors calculate whether you are a normal weight, overweight or obese using a calculation called your body mass index (BMI). It is your weight in kilograms divided by your height squared. A BMI of 18–25kg/m² indicates the normal weight range, BMI 25–30 is overweight, and a BMI of greater than 30 signifies obesity using this measurement. It should be noted that the BMI calculation is based on someone of average build. A muscular body-builder will have a BMI that appears much higher than it should be due to the weight of muscle.

The Weight Set-Point

Your brain will control your weight to a pre-programmed weight set-point. If you lose weight, it will pull it back to your set-point level by decreasing your metabolism (energy used) and increasing your appetite. These processes are very powerful, and your brain will inevitably win any battle if you try to force your weight down by dieting.

Your weight set-point is dependent on:

Genetics – You are much more likely to suffer with obesity if you are from an obese family

Environment – This includes:
- *Your diet*
  - Sugar and refined carbs increase insulin, which blocks the leptin weight-control signal (see above)
  - Fructose*
  - Vegetable oils*
- *Stress (cortisol)* – increases insulin and appetite
- *Sleep (melatonin)* – affects cortisol and appetite
- *Previous dieting* – signals to the brain to store extra energy (fat) in case of future diets

* *The mechanism of how vegetable oils and fructose (fruit sugar) raise a person's weight set-point are explained in chapter 4.*

I asked the students to imagine dieting as a tug of war. On one side is the weight-loss team: dieting (decreased calories) and going to the gym (increased activity). On the other side is

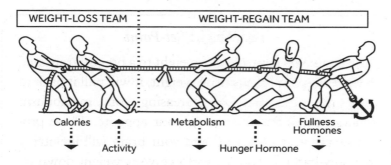

Figure 3: The weight-loss tug of war

the weight-regain team, including decreased metabolism (so you are not burning as much energy), increased hunger and decreased satiety. 'Ultimately, if you try to lose weight, to go away from your set-point through traditional dieting and exercise, the weight-regain team will eventually win.'

The students were intrigued by this explanation of obesity. 'How is a person's weight set-point determined in the first place?' they asked.

'It's a combination of your *genes* and your current *environment*,' I said. 'And by environment, I mean *the type of food you eat, your stress levels* and *your sleep pattern*.'

Your Family

Genetics plays a big role. In fact, it probably accounts for about 70 per cent of where someone's set-point will be. There are lots of studies on identical twins who are brought up in different households. Once they were adults, their weights were compared and all these studies found that their genes contributed around 70 per cent to their weight. This is as you would expect, and when I see patients in clinic they tend to bring relatives who are also

Weight-Loss Plateaus

An interesting observation from many of my patients who have undergone bariatric surgery is their reports of weight-loss stalls. They may notice rapid weight loss for a few weeks or months followed by a plateau in their weight. This can last for a few weeks until suddenly they notice their weight is shifting down again. Often this happens several times on their weight-loss journey. Similar weight-loss plateaus are reported by people who lose a considerable amount of weight by dietary means alone. I think that the explanation for this stepwise weight-loss phenomenon is the ongoing battle between the body's weight-loss and weight-regain teams (as depicted in Figure 3). As weight loss stops and plateaus, there is equal pull between the two teams, so they are at a standstill. But if the weight-loss team continues to pull (as is the case with the powerful changes of surgery), eventually the hypothalamus makes an executive decision – shed some more weight and rebalance. A lighter body needs less energy, meaning there is some spare for more vital functions such as making sure immune defences are intact.

suffering from obesity. And we know that if you are naturally slim you probably also come from a family who have this trait.

Modern Food

But when it comes to having a high set-point, one that is in the overweight or obese range, it is likely that this is caused by a *combination* of those genes with the food environment that you happen to live in and be exposed to. We know that obesity rates are very high in countries that consume the so-called Western diet.* Whereas in countries that avoid Western foods, obesity rates are low. So, if someone has a genetic, or inherited, predisposition to obesity but they stay in a country or area of the world that does not consume Western foods, Asia or Africa for example, then it is likely that they will remain a normal weight. However, if they live in, or move to, a country where it is normal to eat Western food, and that also has the snacking culture of the West, then it is likely that they will start to develop leptin resistance, which will push their weight set-point up.

Bad Environment

It's not just Western food that can cause the weight set-point to increase. Other factors in your surroundings and the way you live can affect it. These include stress and poor sleep. Stress increases the hormone cortisol in the blood. Cortisol causes a survival stress reaction, increasing appetite and blood sugar. In response, more insulin is produced; that insulin blocks the leptin-signalling pathway in the brain; and the resulting leptin resistance causes the set-point to increase and subsequent

---

* The Western diet originated in the US and has been exported around the world. It comprises processed foods (made in factories, with lots of added artificial flavourings, colourings and preservatives), fast food (takeaway food with high levels of refined carbohydrates and cooked in vegetable oils), sweet carbonated drinks (colas) and fruit juices, and both sweet (sugar) and savoury (vegetable oils) snacks. The diet comprises very high levels of sugar, fructose and inflammatory vegetable oils – all factors that can trigger leptin resistance and cause obesity.

weight gain, as your brain instructs your body to reach that new higher set-point by eating more and expending less energy.

Deficiency of Darkness

Many people who live in modern cities are sleep-deprived and this can also shift someone's weight set-point upwards. Melatonin is the hormone produced by the tiny pineal glands at the back of the eyes in response to decreased light. It promotes sleepiness at dusk and helps healthy sleep. Unfortunately, if you live in an environment where there is lots of artificial light, melatonin is not released in significant quantities to promote sleep. Our modern lighting and 24-hour illuminated cities cause a relative deficiency of darkness, and therefore a lack of melatonin.

Melatonin has a secondary effect of decreasing stress and cortisol. If melatonin is deficient (because of a lack of darkness), cortisol levels rise, insulin increases, and again you see a blockage of the leptin hormone in the brain; and because the leptin signal cannot be seen, weight increases along with the person's weight set-point. This is why weight gain commonly occurs after starting shift work, particularly night shifts.

It was time to remove the large part of the stomach that I had stapled. 'Lights on!' I called to my team, and the abdominal skin was once again illuminated brightly by the large overhead operating-theatre lights. I removed one of the large trocars in Mr Johnson's abdomen, and widened the narrow hole in the skin and abdominal wall using a pair of scissors that would not have looked out of place in a kitchen. This was the exciting part of the operation for the students.

'Mother-in-law,'* I said, and Lise handed me a long pole-like grasper with sharp teeth to clench the stomach. I pushed the grasper through the widened hole I had just made – carefully holding my finger in the hole to stop the abdominal gas escaping, and so preserving the space to see inside the abdomen – then grasped the stomach. The narrowest part of the stomach was brought through the hole and finally the students could see directly what the stomach looked like in real life as I eased it gently out.

With a gush of gas the stomach was removed and placed on the kidney-shaped dish that Lise held out ready. By now it was dusky and purple in colour and would resemble a giant shrimp if inflated. 'Please put on some gloves and open up the stomach with those scissors,' I instructed one of the students. This would no doubt be their big story of the week for their family and friends.

As the students enthusiastically opened up the thick muscular wall of the stomach I explained to them exactly how this particular operation would help Mr Johnson. Around 70 per cent of his stomach was about to be discarded, decreasing its capacity. This in itself would mean that he couldn't eat as much and so would lead to some weight loss. 'Normally the body responds to this by increasing appetite, encouraging food-seeking behaviour,' I said. 'But with this operation, those hunger messages are suspended. The part of the stomach that has been removed is responsible for hunger via the special hormone ghrelin, which is secreted from this area. Once this part of the stomach is removed, appetite is also basically

---

* 'Mother-in-law' is a common nickname used for a clawed grasper. It is so named for its scary appearance. Old-fashioned humour still clings on in operating theatres.

removed – depriving the weight-regain team of a key member. For once, the weight-loss team is the winner.'

The operation was finished. I asked Faisal, my highly competent assistant surgeon, to close the skin with sutures, and discarded my gloves and gown in the 'dirty' bin for later incineration. The students had finished their dissection of Mr Johnson's stomach and I had their attention again.

Insurance Policy (Against Future Diets)

'I mentioned that tug of war that goes on when someone tries to lose weight by dieting. It's always the weight-regain team – low metabolism, high appetite, low satiety – that wins in the end. But when you speak to patients in the clinic, they commonly say that not only do they put all their lost weight back on, but they end up being heavier than before they went on the diet. This happens because the brain senses that the environment has become hostile. It senses the calorie restriction that occurred due to the diet and has calculated that this might happen again.'

I then explained that, in caveman times, this might have been because there were previous food shortages, and so the brain would calculate that it wanted the body to carry more energy reserve (fat) around to insure against food shortages in the future. In modern times, where we are lucky enough to live in an era with plentiful food, the same messages are sent to the brain when someone recurrently diets.

'To the brain, diets are the same as recurrent famines, it can't tell the difference. The result: as an insurance policy against future food shortages, it shifts the weight set-point upwards and weight gain follows. So, low-calorie dieting is counterproductive as far as weight loss is concerned. Most patients who end up in the bariatric surgery clinic have tried low-calorie dieting for years or decades, and have eventually concluded that it's just not going to work. They have tried everything and failed every time. This is when they consider bariatric surgery instead.'

'So, what's the best way for someone to lose weight if low-calorie dieting doesn't work?' Wint asked.

The Weight Anchor

I asked them to imagine that a person's weight set-point is like a ship's anchor. 'The ship can try to sail away from the anchor, but it's always eventually stopped. You may be lucky enough for your anchor to be sunk in the "normal weight" area of the sea, but if your anchor is in the "obese" part of the sea, then trying to sail away from that area using force won't work. Imagine that the anchor is attached to the ship with an elasticated rope. The more effort you put into sailing away from your anchor, the stronger the pull of the anchor as the rope stretches. This is what happens if you try to diet and exercise your way to a new weight. The more effort you put in, the more forcefully you will eventually be pulled back into the obese waters.'

Moving Your Weight Anchor

'But,' I continued, 'if you understand how the brain calculates where it wants your body's weight to be – its weight set-point – then you don't have to fight against the anchor by forcibly sailing away from it, i.e. dieting and exercise. You can move the anchor to different waters by changing some of those criteria that the brain is sensing.'

One way the weight anchor can be moved is through dietary

choices. 'Rather than cutting calories, if you change the types of food you eat away from those foods that are going to block the leptin signal, and towards those foods consumed in parts of the world that don't have an obesity problem, you will go some way to shifting the position of your set-point anchor. We know that stopping sugar or going on an ultra-low-carb diet helps people lose weight. But because people are fixated on calories as the ultimate arbiter of weight, they assume that the reason they lose weight during these types of dietary changes is because they are consuming less calories. This is NOT the case. The reason someone loses weight when they cut sugar or reduce carbs is because they no longer need to produce so much insulin. With less insulin, the leptin signal is no longer blocked, and the normal action of leptin resumes, i.e. to stop weight gain by decreasing your desire to eat. By changing your behaviour so that you do not eat these foods, you have in a way upped anchor from the obese part of the sea, sailed some way towards where the healthy ships are moored, and dropped your anchor there. You may not have sailed all the way to normal waters, but you are definitely in healthier waters.'

'So, if all our patients gave up sugar and went low-carb, would they all lose weight and no longer need bariatric surgery?' Wint was playing the role of devil's advocate. Asking the difficult questions for our students' benefit.

'That's a very good point. They would certainly lose some weight. But because they are usually very obese, they also have a great deal of inflammation in their bodies. The inflammation on its own can block leptin signalling, so there will still be leptin resistance present even after lifestyle changes. Also, we have to consider the addictive nature of foods once someone has struggled with obesity for many years. Food companies know that certain foods – particularly sugary and processed foods that have a sugar/oil combination – cause significant feelings of pleasure. This leads to reward-seeking behaviour and eventually habit formation. This type of food becomes a coping mechanism and eventually a form of addiction.

'The craving is not just for food, but for particularly high-calorie foods so that you can refuel as effectively as possible. When you are constantly experiencing these feelings and the food available to you is processed, with colourful labels tempting you, and loaded with sugar and oil, you become a natural target for food companies and end up their victim. Consuming large quantities of Western foods all the time strengthens the reward pathways in your brain and makes it more difficult to give up this food. Habits and addictions are formed. You become a victim of the food environment that you are unfortunate enough to live in. So, yes, in answer to your question, if someone who is severely obese cleans up their eating behaviour they will lose some weight, but they will still have a degree of leptin resistance caused by the inflammation, and this will signal for them to continue eating. Combine these strong hormonal appetite signals with deeply ingrained reward pathways, habits and food addictions, and it's going to be very difficult to continue only eating healthy low-carb, low-sugar foods.

'What most obese people tell me is that their problems really started when they began their *first* diet. They may have only been in the overweight category, and perhaps they wanted to lose weight for an event or to get a summer beach body. As soon as they started trying to force their body, against their brain's will, to a weight lower than their set-point weight, it led to them losing that weight-loss tug of war and eventually becoming heavier than before the diet. Times this by ten, twenty or fifty diets over the years, and eventually their recurrent dieting has forced their weight up so much that they have developed leptin resistance due to the inflammation in their fat and their poor food choices.

'If they had known, when they were young and only slightly overweight, that they could shift their weight downwards by just adjusting the types of foods they eat, and by paying attention to their stress levels and sleep, they would have not needed to go on multiple energy-sapping low-calorie diets over the years. Simple diet and lifestyle adjustments would have been enough for them, and it would have worked. But because most doctors, dieticians and nutritionists don't fully understand obesity, they will still advise calorie restriction to lose weight. Patients are told to try to forcibly sail away from their natural weight anchor, leading to that resistance and rebound, rather than being helped to understand that they need to take up the anchor and sail to healthy waters to permanently lose weight.'

Energy In vs Energy Out

We had talked about how everyone has their own individual weight set-point determined by their genes, their environment (food, stress, sleep) and their previous dietary attempts. And the students now understood why trying to force your body's weight down to below the weight set-point doesn't work. The weight-regain team wins the tug of war. 'Now I want to focus on another area of misunderstanding out there,' I said. 'And that's one of the members of that weight-regain team. I want to explain *metabolism* and how it is the body's ace in the deck to stop weight loss.'

The amount of energy that our bodies use up every day is determined by our metabolism. Metabolism comes in three parts:

Active energy expenditure – This is the amount of energy expended every day in vigorous activity. For most people who don't go to the gym or do a sport, this accounts for only 1–2 per cent of total energy used. Even if you go for a workout it might only account for 10–15 per cent of your energy.

Passive energy expenditure – This is all the energy expended in day-to-day activities such as walking, working in the office, gentle housework or a hobby. It accounts for 20–30 per cent of the total calories a person uses up per day.

Basal metabolism – This is the amount of energy used per day without moving. If you lay in bed all day you would still use this energy. It goes towards all the vital bodily functions that keep you alive, including heart-beat, breathing, heating your body, your immune system, and brain activity. It accounts for around 70 per cent of your total energy expenditure per day. And unlike active and passive energy expenditure, which you have some personal control over, your basal metabolism *cannot* be consciously adjusted. It's out of your control.

So, basal metabolism (which I will call simply *metabolism* from now on) – the amount of energy that we use just to keep our bodies ticking over – accounts for over two-thirds of our total energy expenditure. Anyone who thinks that exercise is the main cause of energy loss is wrong . . . unless you run a half marathon every day, which would use a similar amount of energy to your daily basal metabolism.

Metabolism Is Different for Different People

The main misunderstanding of our metabolism is that it is somehow fixed. Some people might think that they have a very low or a very high metabolism, and that it is set like this long-term. But our metabolism is not stable; it can swing quite dramatically either upwards or downwards, depending on whether our brain is trying to stop us gaining weight or stop us losing weight. Most doctors aren't aware of this, and medical schools still don't teach this. This is why most clinics still adhere to calorie counting and exercise as their weight-loss treatments.

I told the students about a famous experiment that analysed the basal metabolism of ten men who were of similar age, height, weight and build. 'In our conventional understanding of metabolism, we would predict that all ten would have similar metabolisms. We might assume that because they looked the same then the amount of energy they used up via their metabolism would not differ too much. In fact, the difference in metabolism between the highest and the lowest in the group was a staggering 700kcal per day. This amount of energy is the same as that used up during a 10k run, or consumed in a large three-course meal. Many similar studies have found the same – that metabolism differs drastically between individuals.

'But we also know that not only does metabolism differ between different people, but that it can fluctuate upwards or downwards in the same person in response to their environment. This is where understanding the weight anchor is important. The brain uses metabolism to try to keep your weight at around the level of your weight set-point. It is acting like the elasticated rope in our anchor analogy.'

Power-Saving Mode

I then gave an example. 'You want to lose weight for an upcoming event, maybe a wedding or a holiday. You do this by cutting your calories from maybe 2,000kcal per day to around 1,500kcal. At first you notice that you do indeed lose some weight. However, in a similar way to your smartphone sensing that its power is running down and switching to power-saving mode, after a short period of time your body will sense your weight loss and adapt to your decreased calorie intake by turning down your metabolism by the same amount that you have been calorie-restricting. Human power-saving mode is activated, saving 500kcal per day, and you will see that despite continuing to calorie-restrict, your scales are no longer shifting. Your body has adapted to your diet.'

The Human Dimmer Switch

'Imagine your metabolism as being like a dimmer switch on a lamp. Your body can easily turn that dimmer switch down. Things are still functioning but less energy is being used. The reason that your metabolic dimmer switch is turned down is that the brain senses that your body has lost weight and is veering away from your weight anchor. Your brain utilizes a dimming of your metabolism, plus an increased appetite and decreased satiety to pull your weight back towards your weight anchor.

'Interestingly, changes to your metabolism can also protect you against *gaining* too much weight. Most people, when they are not consciously dieting, eat more food than they need. In order to stop you storing those excess calories and gaining excessive weight, your metabolism adapts to overeating by *increasing* the energy you expend. The dimmer switch is turned up to bright and your weight remains the same. Just as you increase calorie intake, so your body increases the amount of energy you use up, preventing too much weight gain away from your natural weight anchor. This explains that annoying friend or colleague you might have who seems to be able to eat and eat but never puts on weight.'

Metabolism Changes Dramatically

Our resting (or basal) metabolism accounts for 70 per cent of the energy we use up per day. It is the energy used by us for vital internal functions such as heating our bodies, our heartbeat, breathing, using our brain to think and calculate, and our protective immune system.

The amount of energy used up by our resting metabolism can vary by up to 700kcal per day. This is the same amount of energy that is required to do a hard workout in the gym for over one hour, or the same amount of calories consumed in a large meal.

When our brain senses our weight is too low, it will switch our resting metabolism down to save energy. When our brain thinks our weight is too high, it will increase our metabolism to help weight loss.

I was concluding the teaching session now. 'And these are the reasons that Mr Johnson could not lose weight – his genes combined with living in a country where the diet is high in sugar, refined carbs and vegetable oils. This means that his insulin levels need to be high to cope with the diet. The insulin in turn blocks that fat hormone leptin, which is supposed to signal to his brain when he's carrying too much weight. With leptin blocked, his brain can't see the fat, and is in fact getting starvation messages. His weight anchor shifts upwards. And when he tries to lose the weight by dieting and exercise, his metabolic dimmer switch is turned down, meaning that his body adapts itself to the diet and the diet fails.'

Our medical students were nodding enthusiastically. I hoped that their newfound knowledge of obesity would make them more compassionate when treating people struggling with it in their long future careers, whatever branch of medicine they chose to pursue.

I turned to Wint, who was in the process of waking Mr Johnson up. He had now been transferred to his extra-large hospital bed and was in the process of coughing out his breathing tube. 'Operation is over, Mr Johnson, everything went OK, just relax.' It was time for coffee.

CHAPTER 2

The Modern Kitchen

Understanding Our Eating Environment

'Food is the place where you begin.'

Vandana Shiva

We learned in the previous chapter how our weight anchor can be influenced by the types of foods that we eat. If we consume a diet that is too full of sugar and refined carbohydrates, it will increase our insulin levels and that insulin can block our natural weight sensor – the hormone leptin. The brain gets confused by this and we gain weight. It's the same with foods containing too much vegetable oil and too much of the fruit sugar fructose. They also cause a misfiring of weight-control signals and lead to weight gain. Contrary to most people's understanding of their diet, it's not the amount of calories in these foods that cause weight gain, it's how they disrupt our weight-control signalling.

In the last forty years, much of the food that is available to us has become full of sugar, refined carbs, sweet fructose sugar and artificial vegetable oils – just the types of foods that make our weight-control signalling misfire. Processed foods now account for 56 per cent of the total calories consumed per day by the average UK citizen. The figure is even higher in the USA. In the same forty-year period, obesity rates in the UK have increased from around 5–10 per cent of the population to the current level of between a quarter and a third of the population.

But processed food doesn't just cause obesity, it is also responsible for many other health conditions that only affect so-called affluent countries. As I will explain, modern foods are causing modern diseases.

In this chapter (and the next), we will take a deep dive into food processing and how ultra-processed foods (UPFs) impact our brains and our bodies. Once we are clear in our minds how dangerous these foods are, we can identify easier ways to defend ourselves against their ill effects, without resorting to willpower alone. The more we understand, the less willpower is required to develop healthy habits.

January 2040, Your Kitchen in the Future

Imagine for a moment the ultimate in revolutionary home cooking . . . the ability to make your favourite supermarket snacks in your own home from basic ingredients. It's the best of both worlds – spending a mindful hour or so in your large, brightly lit and ultra-modern kitchen, listening to your favourite tracks on Alexa while preparing a tasty snack for when your friends visit.

Our modern kitchen of the future needs to be fully stocked with basic ingredients. Fortunately, there are only a handful of items needed to make most snacks. Sugar, flour (wheat, corn, rice, potato), starch powder (from corn or potato), vegetable oils (sunflower, rapeseed, palm, saffron), cocoa and sugar.

We need some great new cooking instruments in our futuristic kitchen (that's why it's in the future, as they haven't yet been invented). A kitchen-sized industrial press and roller to squash and squeeze our snacks into cute shapes; an ultra-high-powered mixer to make sure of a perfect blend; and a powerful centrifuge to filter out dirt and debris. We are going to need a red-hot steamer, and a high-speed hot-air oven or precision oil fryer, depending on what we are cooking. Finally, a cool spray machine to coat our snacks with delicious powders once they are cooked.

To make things safe, we need to invest in a couple more machines. For our crisp recipes, we are going to need an electroporation machine, which puts little holes in the chips and stops cancerous acrylamide forming.* And before our food is ready to serve, we're going to have to pass it through an X-ray scanner to ensure that no plastic, glass, bone or stones have got into it . . . we don't want an awkward situation when a friend breaks a tooth.

The Long 'Spice' Rack

We need to make our snacks taste just like the real thing, so there is a section of the kitchen dedicated to flavour enhancers. These include preservatives and antioxidants (to stop them going off), thickeners and sweeteners – and of course, most importantly, sections for flavour enhancement and colouring.

Flavour and colour are going to be important in our finished product. We can make our snacks into wonderful shapes and interesting crunchy or chewy textures using our new cooking machines, but they will all be a drab and unappetizing brown or grey in colour (imagine seeing your food through a

---

* Acrylamide is a white, water-soluble chemical that is produced as a by-product of cooking at high temperatures foods that contain asparagine (a protein amino acid) and glucose. It is associated with an increased risk of developing cancer.

black-and-white filter) and probably won't taste that interesting. If you lost your taste after a Covid infection you will understand the importance of this. We don't want the finished product to be grey and foul-tasting, so a sprinkling of flavour and a dash of colour are essential. Our guests (and many other mammals and birds) have evolved to see bright-coloured fruits as an 'eat me' signal from plants. That's why we love to eat golden, brightly coloured foods (think baked beans), so those food dyes are essential for the preparation of our palates.

This area of our modern kitchen will be our E-number section. We could have a large rack of tiny jars, just like the spice section in the supermarket, but with each jar containing different coloured powders and oils labelled with their E-number. The whole back wall of your kitchen might contain these racks, with the jars arranged in order – E100–199 Colours, E200–299 Preservatives, E300–399 Antioxidants . . . all the way to E1000–1599 Additional additives . . . Altogether 319 E-number jars in total . . . we are going to need a long spice rack.

Before we start cooking we need to ensure our food is safe, so we are going to take some of the E-numbers out of our rack. We need the foods to be OK for all our friends and wouldn't want to give them anything banned in their own country or maybe potentially dangerous for their health. So we are going to start by removing some of the colourings. Let's get rid of the 'Southampton Six' first.* These are: E102

---

* The Southampton Six are a group of six food colouring additives identified as potentially causing hyperactivity in children when mixed with sodium benzoate (E211, a preserving and flavouring element found in snacks, fruit juices, condiments and pickles). Many are banned in Scandinavian countries. The UK food safety agency asked the food industry to voluntary withdraw these food colourings.

Tarazine, a yellow dye originating from petroleum (associated with ADHD and cancer); E104 Quinoline Yellow, a green-yellow dye originating from coal tar (suspected link to ADHD in children); E129 Allura Red, or 'Red 40', made from petroleum and in many fruit bars, cereals, cake mixes, flavoured milk, red-coloured drinks and gummies (causes allergic reactions); E124 Ponceu R4, a strawberry-red food colouring (cancer risk in animals, unknown in humans); E110 Sunset Yellow, made from petroleum (suspected ADHD links); and E122 Azorubine, a solid red dye made from petrol, which is used in make-up and in some cheeses and dried fruits (it contains beta-naphthylamine and is associated with potential cancer risk). We should probably also put E220 (sulphur dioxide) to one side too, as it can make asthma much worse.

I'm going to make my food colouring easy by creating my own easel of favourite colours, as if I were painting a masterpiece in oils:

GREEN – E141 copper and chlorophyll

BRILLIANT BLUE – E133 from coal tar

ORANGE/YELLOW – E100 from turmeric

RED – E120 from egg yolk and dried insects

BLACK – E151 from coal tar

OK, now the big decision . . . what special treats to create to impress my friends so they will keep coming back for more?

I'm going to prepare a savoury snack, maybe a cracker or a crazy-looking crisp they just won't be able to get enough of, and a colourful and flavoursome drink to perk them up.

The Addictive Crisp-like Snack

INGREDIENTS

Basic
    Potato flour
    Corn flour
    Rice flour
    Corn starch
    Wheat starch
    Vegetable oil (rapeseed)

Flavour enhancers
    E631 disodium inosinate (from meat/chicken waste products)
    E1400 maldrexin (starch texture enhancer for improved 'mouthfeel')
    E627 disodium guanylate (from dried seaweed)
    E621 monosodium glutamate (from bacterial fermentation)
    Salt

Emulsifiers
    E471 mono- and diglycerides
    E414 gum arabic (from tree bark, popular in watercolour painting)

Anti-caking agent
    E551 silicon dioxide (sand)

Preservative
    E220 sulphur dioxide (antifungal, but also eliminates vitamin E)

Colours
    E100 orange/yellow
    E120 red

PREPARATION

Get all your ingredients ready – the large canisters of flour and all the E-numbers you are going to use should be within easy reach.

You are not going to need a chopping board or knife to prepare these snacks, so store these away and get out your scales and ultra-high-powered mixer.

Fill your precision oil fryer with vegetable oil and switch it on to high so that there is time for the fat to reach the required temperature.

Fill a mixing bowl with the potato, corn and rice flour, the corn starch and wheat starch. Add pinches from pots E631, E1400, E627 and E621 (for flavour), emulsify with a touch of E471 and E414, sprinkle in some sand (E551) and add salt to taste. Protect the final product from going off (for months) with E220. Finally, colourings E100 and E120 should be infused until the colour is a golden orange.

Add water and knead, until the mixture becomes solid but not too moist. Place in the ultra-high-powered mixer, take a step back (it's very loud and vibrates a lot) and turn on for two minutes.

Turn on your industrial roller and set it to 2mm. Attach to your shaper and turn the setting to oval lattice (size 5cm x 3cm).

Take your mixture from the ultra-high-powered mixer and push it through the roller. When the oval lattices appear from the shaper, place them individually onto a slightly curved deep frying basket and submerge them in the precision oil fryer for ten seconds exactly.

Leave to cool off in a separate corner of the kitchen.

COATING

Once the crisps are dry, use the spray machine to splash them with liquid smoke (from the condensation of smoke) and paprika powder.

PACKAGING

The kitchen of the future will have its own packaging machines, including one for stackable crisps like these. The tubes will be brightly coloured (I'm going for a red one but the choice is yours) and you can add your own health labels onto them. For this one I'm adding 'NO SATURATED FAT and NO ADDED SUGAR'.

Stack the crisps into the tube containers until full and close them with the sealing machine.

That's it. Job complete, and snacks ready and stored.

January 2041 – Your Party

The great thing about your snack is that, thanks to the preservative that you added (E220), it can keep for a long time. A whole year has passed, and your friends are about to arrive for a party. You have also managed to save a sweet, chewy colourful candy that you prepared, plus a variety of very colourful sweet drinks (green, blue, yellow, orange and red).

As your friends arrive and make themselves comfortable, you dash down to the cellar (where you stored your crisps last year), dust off the cobwebs from the carton to make them presentable, and distribute them.

They certainly look good on the plate – an attractive deep orange colour. As your friends eat them they experience a pleasant crunching sensation, followed by a nice slightly gummy mouthfeel from E414, and a soft texture provided by E1400. The tastes of protein from E621, sugary starch, salt, and the hint of paprika excite them as the reward pathways in their brains light up. The sweetness is accentuated by the sugar-laden soft drinks you have laid on. The atmosphere of the party livens up as your friends all experience simultaneous pleasant feelings. 'Nice flavour!' . . . 'beautiful texture' . . . 'these crisps are so more-ish I must get the recipe' are just some of the compliments for the chef.

As the contents of your creation are absorbed into your friends' bodies (apart from the sand), digestive reactions start, the starches create a glucose spike and a large amount of insulin is required to deal with the onslaught. The insulin blocks the fat-fullness signal from leptin and your friends remain hungry. The vegetable oils release vast quantities of omega-6 into their bloodstreams, covering their cells, causing inflammation and slowing their metabolism. The fructose in the drinks triggers the breakdown of the cells' energy currency and gives the feeling of starvation, making your friends hungry. The various E-numbers ping around their bodies and brains, creating as-yet-unknown consequences. Unfortunately, no one has consumed anything of nutritional value so far.

A Brief History of Processed Foods

What is processed food? Isn't all food (except for a fruit picked directly from a tree) processed in some way? How can we define one food as processed and another as not processed? As with so many issues around our food, this question is confusing. The answer is that yes, most of the food that we eat has in some way been processed, but it is the *amount* of processing that goes into making a food that seems to matter to our health.

Throughout history humans have been ingenious enough to change and manipulate raw foods to make them:

Easier to chew and digest
Taste better*
Last longer without spoiling

Food processing began 200,000 years ago, when early humans discovered how to make and control fire. Early humans were able to cook meat by roasting it (tenderizing it and making it easier to chew), and to bake previously indigestible energy-rich tubers (sweet potato, cassava, etc.) to make them more digestible. With the advent of agriculture 12,000 years ago, humans discovered that pounding grains and mixing them with water and yeast could make bread, which quickly became an essential food – easy to transport and relatively resistant to spoiling.

Then, 5,000 years ago, a new drink was discovered in Persia, made from the fermentation of barley. Beer became a common drink mainly because of its valuable calorie content and its stability. Early beer had a low alcohol content, so it was difficult to become inebriated even if it was drunk all day. The alcohol content meant it was resistant to harbouring disease-causing bacteria, unlike stored water, which could spoil. The slaves that built the Pyramids of Giza in Egypt were given a daily ration of at least five litres of beer to sustain them (and possibly lift their spirits).

Around the same time, fermented cow and goat milk was used to make cheeses and yogurt. These foods had a much lower lactose content than milk, making them easier to digest,

---

* Cooking is a form of food processing that is designed to make food tastier and more digestible.

and could be stored for much longer than milk, which before refrigeration would spoil rapidly.

Then, around 1,500 years ago in India, a big milestone in human food history was reached . . . sugar was produced for the first time. The food that would, generations later, contribute so much pleasure and at the same time so much ill health was extracted from sugar-cane juice through presses, boiled, and then dried to make sugar granules. This easily transportable commodity was used to produce a wide range of sweets, particularly in the Middle East (it was named 'white gold' by English crusaders). Sugar plantations were built by European countries in the Caribbean – worked by slaves – making the commodity cheaper and more widely available.

How Food Spoils and How to Prevent It

Fresh foods tend to spoil, or become rancid, giving them an unpleasant smell and taste if left for too long. This is due to two main processes: oxidation (think of an apple going brown) and the overgrowth of bacteria or yeast (think of mouldy bread). Throughout the ages, we have invented ingenious ways to protect foods from becoming stale or rotten and help them last longer. Today, we would say to 'increase their shelf life'.

DRYING

Drying fruits helps stop spoilage by increasing their concentration of sugar and creating an inhospitable environment for bacteria. This method of processing was popular in ancient Rome. Drying meat to preserve it for later use – such as in a food-scarce winter – has been used for thousands of years.

CURING

The use of spices to enhance the flavour of meat and help preserve it was introduced by ancient Indian civilizations. Known in the West as 'currying' (from the Tamil word *kari*, a spiced sauce used in South Indian cooking), curing meat by coating it with a combination of salt, sugar and spices helps draw out the moisture and stops bacteria growing. In addition, it improves the meat's flavour.

SALTING

Salting food, particularly meat and fish, dates back to the ancient Greeks and Egyptians. It works by limiting the amount of water available to bacteria, reducing their spread and preventing spoiling. Like many other preserving techniques, it also enhances the flavour of the food.

SMOKING

Smoking also goes back to ancient European civilizations and indigenous North American tribes. By smoking meat or fish for an extended period of time, bacteria are killed. Smoking also adds a distinctive flavour to food.

PICKLING

Pickling in vinegar, salt water (brine) or alcohol prevents bacteria growing by creating a hostile acidic environment. Cabbage can be preserved for long periods of time by the process of fermentation,* creating acids that help protect from spoiling and add distinctive flavours. Kimchi, originating in

---

* Fermentation is a process where microorganisms (bacteria and yeast) break down the energy-containing carbon bonds in food without the need for oxygen. The by-product of the process is the formation of alcohol.

Korea, and sauerkraut, from Germany, are popular examples of this process.

TINNING

In the late eighteenth century, Napoleon Bonaparte offered a prize for the invention of a process that could preserve food for longer so that it could be supplied to his far-flung armies. The prize of 12,000 francs was won by the discovery that heating food inside sealed containers could preserve the contents. Food (initially corned beef) was cooked and then packed inside sealed cans, and the cans were then heated to a high temperature to kill any remaining bacteria in the food. This method ensured food remained edible for long periods of time, opening up the possibility of worldwide export and distribution. In the nineteenth century, tinned foods became an important global commodity.

Since the 1940s, vacuum packaging (think of the airtight plastic wrapping around the salmon products in your supermarket food aisle) has become common. It works by completely removing the oxygen from around the food. The atmospheric vacuum created means that the fats in the food do not oxidize and become rancid as quickly. This advance in technology means the food's shelf life can be extended without the necessity to alter the food (by drying, boiling or salting).

LIFE SUPPORT FOR LETTUCES

You may have noticed that much of the vegetable section in your local supermarket contains products within plastic packaging. Despite the pollution that this causes, the packaging keeps leafy vegetables fresher for longer by changing the atmosphere within it. Unlike animals, who stop breathing when they die, freshly cut vegetables such as lettuce or broccoli continue to breathe. If the atmosphere around the plant includes high levels of their favourite food – carbon dioxide – they will stay fresher for longer. Your standard gas-filled plastic bag of lettuce leaves in the supermarket has been infused with lethal levels of carbon dioxide for us (5 per cent), but this is abundant food for the lettuce. This method of prolonging fresh foods' shelf life is called modified atmosphere packaging.

COOLING

In the 1950s, refrigeration and freezing of food in the home became common. Bacteria love a temperature of 37 °C (the same as a human body) to flourish, and therefore storing food at a lower temperature helps it withstand bacterial invasion and prolongs the time before it spoils.

The Evolution of Modern Food

As we've seen, historically food processing was for the purpose of making food easier to chew and digest, and to last longer without spoiling, with the added bonus that sometimes these processes could make the food taste better. But over the last fifty years the rationale for food processing changed. As technology to keep foods fresher for longer (by using chemical additives) advanced, so international food companies saw an opportunity. Foods could be packaged and exported to far-flung corners of the world without the risk that they would spoil. Convenience-store keepers and supermarket-owners love this type of product, as the food remains edible for months or years and therefore keeps its value until it is sold. Consumers (such as me and you) find foods that do not go off convenient – they can be stored in the pantry until required, and this is particularly important in the developing world, where fridges and freezers may not be readily available. And, most importantly, the food manufacturers love these products. The core ingredients – such as flour, sugar, salt and vegetable oils – are cheap to buy, and when the food is made on an industrial scale it is cheap to produce, meaning huge profit margins for these new processed foods – profits that far outstrip fresh foods. Instead of food processing being for our benefit, as it historically had been, it became a way to make a lot of money.

Modern Preserving Techniques

More recently, foods have had their shelf life prolonged by the addition of chemicals. Without these additives, modern processed foods are just as susceptible to spoiling, if left, as fresh meat, fish or vegetables. The process is the same – either they will spoil because of bacterial overgrowth, making them dangerous to eat, or they will turn rancid because the fats and oils within them have become oxidized. Food chemical additives can either be antimicrobial, limiting the growth of bacteria and fungi, or act as antioxidants, limiting the oxygenation of the food.

CHEMICAL ANTIMICROBIALS

Common antimicrobial additives in modern foods include calcium propionate, sodium nitrate (and nitrite) and sulphites. Calcium propionate (E282) is used in baked products and other processed foods. It works by releasing acid into the food, and the acidic environment means that bacteria cannot grow as easily. The side effects of too much calcium propionate include digestive problems such as bloating and diarrhoea. There is some concern that it can cause ADHD in children and it has been linked to autism in animal studies.

Sodium nitrates are used in fertilizers and to make explosives; they are also found abundantly in plants. However, although we take in sodium nitrate when we eat vegetables, when they are artificially added to processed and cured meats, they lead to an increased risk of colon cancer in the future.

Sulphur dioxide (E220), which is derived from sulphuric acid, is used on dried fruits for both antibacterial and antioxidant properties, ensuring that the fruit retains its colourful appearance. This and other sulphites (E220–E228)* are used as antifungal and antibacterial agents in many foods.† It is accepted that the presence of sulphite preservatives – on or inside food – can cause autoimmune and other reactions, including asthma, rashes, itchy skin, flushing, abdominal cramps and diarrhoea. It has also been reported that sulphites adversely affect the sensitive balance of the microbes that live in our guts (the microbiome), leading to unknown consequences.

CHEMICAL ANTIOXIDANTS

Butylated hydroxyanisole (E320) and butylated hydroxytoluene (E321) are petrochemicals that are added to food to attract and soak up oxygen molecules. When oxygen reacts with oils (particularly the unhealthy vegetable oils that are found in many processed foods), a reaction occurs causing the release of foul-smelling gases such as aldehydes and ketones. This makes the oil or the food containing the oil smell like aged cheese, a

---

* E220 sulphur dioxide, E221 sodium sulphite, E222 sodium bisulphite, E223 sodium metabisulphite, E226 calcium sulphite, E227 calcium bisulphite, E228 potassium bisulphite.

† Sulphites are used as preserving agents in drinks (cordials, wine, fruit juices, soft drinks), biscuits, bread, pizza dough, dried potato, gravy granules, sauces, fruit toppings and prawns.

process called rancidification . . . it smells 'off'. By soaking up roaming oxygen, the butylates delay this process.

As well as being antioxidant food additives, they are used in cosmetics, commercial lubrication oils, jet fuel and as embalming agents. Unfortunately, despite these chemicals being present in many common food items that may inhabit your fridge and pantry, they have been officially recognized by the US National Institute of Health as carcinogenic (the medical term for causing cancer). Despite numerous animal studies linking butylate ingestion to the risk of skin cancers, they are still licensed as safe in most parts of the world due to their low dose in most processed foods. The state of California is an exception: its public health authorities have listed butylates as carcinogenic in humans.

One of these antioxidants, called butylhydroquinone (TBHQ, E319) is even more startling. As Michael Pollen wrote in his book *The Omnivore's Dilemma* of its use in Chicken McNuggets, it 'is either sprayed directly on the nugget or the inside of the box it comes in to "help preserve freshness". According to *A Consumer's Dictionary of Food Additives*, TBHQ is a form of butane (i.e. lighter fluid) the FDA allows processors to use sparingly in our food: It can comprise no more than 0.02 percent of the oil in a nugget. Which is probably just as well, considering that ingesting a single gram of TBHQ can cause "nausea, vomiting, ringing in the ears, delirium, a sense of suffocation, and collapse". Ingesting five grams of TBHQ can kill.'

Know Your Enemy (or Customer)

According to a 2021 report, the global processed food market generates revenues of $2.3 trillion per year. In order to make their vast profits, food companies have looked to maximize sales by making their food irresistible to customers. They need to attract us to their product and make us want to go back and purchase it again and again. To do this, they have employed thousands of food scientists to study what humans (yes, that's me and you again) enjoy the most about food. They have identified several key factors that we love when choosing food, tasting it, chewing it and consuming it.

TASTE COMBINATION

Like all animals, humans can sense whether something might be edible or inedible by its smell and taste, and by how it looks and feels. We have five built-in sensors on our tongue that can sense sweetness, sourness, saltiness, bitterness and umami (a protein-like taste). A combination of salt, sugar and umami is the perfect taste for us. Umami – the taste we would normally experience when we eat meat – can be artificially produced by adding monosodium glutamate (MSG, E621) and 5' nitrates (disodium 5'-ribonucleotides, E635). Salt always improves the pleasure of sugary foods. Food scientists have determined that the ideal additive proportion is 1–1.5 per cent salt, 0.15 per cent MSG, and 0.02 per cent nitrates. This makes the most addictive taste.

MOUTHFEEL

When the food is within our mouths, as well as stimulating our taste buds it gives us the sensation of how it feels and what consistency it has. This is called mouthfeel. Whereas taste imparts 10 per cent of the sensation of food, mouthfeel contributes more than 40 per cent. The two most important factors in mouthfeel are *dynamic contrast* and *mouth coating*.

Crunchiness, chewiness, slipperiness, temperature (hot, cold or lukewarm) and spiciness are examples of how the food is sensed as you chew it. If a food has many different elements of mouthfeel, such as crunchiness, gumminess or spiciness, these different combinations make the food more desirable – this is dynamic contrast.

The second, and probably most important part of mouthfeel is mouth coating. This occurs when a food is in an emulsion (a combination of watery and fatty foods mixed together). Emulsions give a highly desirable 'melting' sensation in the mouth – examples include butter, ice cream, chocolate, and many different sauces and dressings such as mayonnaise or salad dressings.

BRIGHT COLOURS

We love food to be brightly coloured. From an evolutionary perspective, edible fruits developed bright colours to attract animals to eat them and distribute their seeds. We (as animals ourselves) find beige or grey foods unappetizing compared to brighter-coloured options. Unfortunately, beige or grey is the natural colour of highly processed foods, and this is why they need food colourings to be added to make them look more palatable, so that people will buy them. Just as the dynamic contrast of different mouth sensations (crunchy, chewy, etc.) is desirable, when different bright colours light up our food they also become more appetizing. This is the reason that cakes are decorated with different brightly coloured creams or sprinkles, and why fast-food restaurants add contrasting ingredients of coloured lettuce, tomato and cheese to their burgers, making them look irresistible on that billboard ad. Michelin-starred chefs know this too, and the combination of different mouthfeels and different colours in their signature dishes makes consuming them a particularly pleasant and mindful experience (until the bill arrives of course).

CALORIE DENSITY

The calorie density of a food is the number of calories (units of energy) packed into it, measured as calories per gram. When we eat a food, our stomach and intestine sense the number of calories it contains and send messages to our brains relaying this information. Water has a calorie density of zero, and fat (such as butter) has the highest calorie density at 9kcal/g. Experiments have revealed that a calorie density of 4–5kcal/g is the most desirable for us when it comes to the foods we eat. Not surprisingly, most modern processed foods have a calorie density of 4–5.

THE FOOD PLEASURE EQUATION

The final calculation when producing a new food is a combination of all of the factors described above:

Taste + colour + mouthfeel + mouth coating + calorie density = ultimate desirability and addictiveness

If a food is lower in calorie density than the optimal 4–5kcal/g, then extra colours, mouthfeel and tastes need to be added to make up for this. Think crunchy, flavoured and coloured popcorn – what is lost in calories is compensated for in taste sensations.

Hedonic Taste Code

So, thanks to many years of research and thousands of tasting experiments involving human volunteers, food scientists have been able to gauge the pleasure we experience from differing foods. This is our hedonic taste code. Through painstaking research, they have discovered exactly how our taste code works. What foods we want the most, what foods we crave, what foods we go back to again and again. It's as if our precious, and previously secret, taste code has been hacked, leaving us vulnerable to those that have this precious data.

Using this data, our clever food scientists have been able to invent new foods that are hyper-palatable to us. Foods that tend to be made from the similar ingredients of sugar, flour, unhealthy oils and salt, and are therefore cheap and low in nutritional quality. Foods that tend to be craved and overeaten.

Our taste code is the very foundation of our food choice, embedded within us to help us survive. Now food companies have gained knowledge of it, we are no longer fully in charge of what we eat.

In the real world, by which I mean the world of real food, the perfect hedonic and pleasurable food does not exist. Perhaps the best effort that nature has produced are our brightly coloured and sweet fresh fruits. But thanks to modern manufactured foods, we now have a daily choice of the most beautifully pleasurable foods. These might be fast foods, such as crispy, salty, umami, chewy fried chicken, or a hamburger stacked with different-coloured layers (bun, lettuce, tomato, cheese, burger) in bright, desirable combinations and different-tasting layers (sweet bun, burger, ketchup, sticky cheese). Or the sweet spot for our food pleasure could be mass-produced sweet or savoury snacks – the brightly packaged food items that can be found in the middle section of supermarkets. Many of these food packages have labels claiming the positive health and nutritional qualities of the food: added vitamins, fat-free, no added sugar, heart-healthy, vegan-friendly, etc. But what are the real health consequences of our modern designer foods?

Food nutritionists study the health effects of different types of foods, telling us what to eat and what not to eat. They tend to break down food into different parts. They might analyse the cholesterol content for instance, or the salt content, or they might concentrate on a particular type of vitamin or mineral. They analyse how much of one nutritional component of a food is eaten by people, and then take a look at whether the people consuming a lot of it are healthier or sicker. Whether they die early or live longer and healthier lives.

This type of population research is what much of our food advice is based upon. However, these studies are notoriously unreliable and inaccurate. This is the reason that food advice is constantly changing depending on the latest (usually inaccurate) study. One week, eggs are terribly dangerous to eat, the next week they are good for us. The advice of nutritionists confuses us. By breaking foods down into individual components, they blur the line between more natural fresh foods and processed foods. This is called food reductionism. It plays into the hands of the food industry, which looks at the latest nutritional research and adds or subtracts elements depending on the current advice. It can then advertise these changes (low-fat, low-sugar, low-calorie) to help drive sales. The poor isolated fresh and natural foods have no such advantages. Fruits can't be labelled 'low-cholesterol' and meat can't have a 'no added sugar' sticker on it, as this would look ridiculous. We know these foods, and we know what's in them.

When people start to eat more processed food, they risk becoming obese and are more likely to develop obesity-related diseases such as diabetes or high blood pressure. In addition, people, or populations of people, who consume lots of this type of food tend to be unwell with other 'modern' diseases: inflammatory or autoimmune conditions such as heart disease, arthritis, asthma and colitis. Or newer diseases that are becoming more and more common, such as painful fibromyalgia or IBS or Alzheimer's. Modern food seems to cause modern diseases.

The problem for scientists has been proving that these conditions are related to processed food. The lawyers of the food industry will point out that most food (as we have seen) is processed in some way. Nutritionists focus only on a particular element of a food, reducing both fresh and processed foods to their base elements and muddling the differences between them. They say cholesterol, or saturated fat, or salt or sugar are bad for us, and that we should cut down on the foods containing too much of them. However, this ignores whether the food is natural or if it has been highly processed. They will not mind if it is a designer food, bringing together many ingredients, preservatives, colourings and flavourings. It won't matter that it is mass-produced in factories and dressed in brightly coloured packages with health labels signalling it is good for you. Exported around the world, this food will sit on supermarket shelves for months before catching the eye of the unwary, vulnerable people whose food code has been hacked. But does this food really cause them to become sick?

How Much Is Too Much Food Processing?

The confusion over food reductionism and food processing was highlighted in the early 2000s by Carlos Monteiro, a Brazilian doctor and scientist with an interest in the nutritional health of the population. Brazilians are traditionally proud of their health and fitness, but Monteiro noted that the number of young Brazilians with obesity had more than doubled in ten years, going from 7.5 per cent in 2002 to 17.5 per cent in 2013.

The paradox was that people were buying *less* sugar in this time. However, when he analysed the population's food habits in more detail, he found that although they were buying less sugar and using less of it to cook and bake in their kitchens, the total amount of sugar that they were consuming had increased significantly. The source of this sugar was processed foods. The population were cooking and baking less and consuming ready-made processed foods more, with an apparent detrimental effect on their health.

He noted that traditional government advice on healthy eating was based upon the *food pyramid*. The original US Department of Agriculture (USDA) food pyramid of 1992 describes the foods that should be eaten the most at the bottom, including 'complex' carbohydrates such as unrefined (i.e. wholegrain) pasta, wheat and rice. Above this is the section for fruit and vegetables (3–5 servings). Getting towards the top of the pyramid are meat, fish and dairy products (2–3 servings). The point of the pyramid is fats, oils and sweets (use sparingly). But Monteiro noted that much of the food that was being consumed by the population was not included in the pyramid, as it was ultra-processed or highly refined. People were ignoring the government eating advice. 'It's time to demolish the pyramid,' he wrote in 2011. Shortly afterwards, the Brazilian government, taking Monteiro's advice, did just that. They introduced a completely new concept of classifying foods, to highlight to people that ultra-processed foods are bad for them and that home-cooked fresh foods will keep them healthy. With their new system – called NOVA (after a new star) – they precisely defined what types of food should be avoided. It is worth looking at the NOVA system in more detail to gain a greater understanding of processed foods.

The NOVA Classification

NOVA divides foods into four categories.

Group 1 NOVA foods are *unprocessed or minimally processed foods*. Unprocessed foods are direct from nature: vegetables, fruits, animal meat and fish. Minimally processed foods include those that have been dried, pasteurized or frozen. Examples include fresh or frozen fruits or vegetables, wholegrain rice, grits (including buckwheat), eggs, legumes (lentils, chickpeas, etc.), unsalted nuts, milk, yogurt, fresh or frozen meat and fish, fresh or dried cut herbs and spices, tea and fresh coffee.

Group 2 NOVA foods are the ingredients that are used in the kitchen to help cook and flavour the fresh foods of Group 1. These include salt, sugar, flour and oils. This group of foods is classified as *processed culinary ingredients*.

Group 3 is termed *processed foods* and includes natural foods that appear in Group 1 that have been processed to help preserve them, usually industrially, by using ingredients from Group 2 foods such as salt, sugar or oil. Foods that have been pickled, salted, fermented or canned fall into this group, as well as traditionally made bread such as sourdough (made with unrefined wheat flour, yeast, water and salt only). Examples of foods in this group include cheese, ham, canned vegetables and pulses, canned fish such as sardines, salted nuts, preserved meats (salted, dried or cured), and fermented alcoholic drinks such as beer and wine.

Group 4 of the NOVA food classification system is *ultra-processed foods* (UPFs). These foods use many of the ingredients in Group 2 (processed culinary ingredients) such as salt, sugar, oils and flour. But instead of using these ingredients sparingly to make Group 1 ingredients taste better, as a chef would use them in a kitchen, they are used in large quantities and

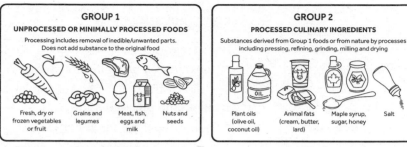

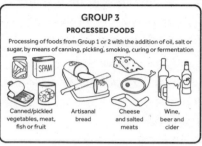

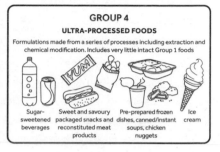

Figure 4: The NOVA food classification system

combined with artificial flavourings, emulsifiers and colourings, ingredients unfamiliar to a non-industrial kitchen, to make them highly palatable. This modern food is aggressively marketed, and is highly profitable due to cheap ingredients. Because UPFs are so convenient they can be consumed anytime and anywhere, and often will replace freshly made meals.

Monteiro wrote that this group of foods contains 'formulations of ingredients, mostly of exclusively industrial use, typically created by a series of industrial techniques and processes'. These foods tend to be energy-dense and nutritionally unbalanced.

Examples of ultra-processed foods include breakfast cereals and bars, packaged breads, chicken nuggets, fish fingers, burgers, hot dogs, pre-prepared pizza and pasta, pastries, cakes, margarines and spreads, instant noodles, powdered soups, sweetened yogurts, sweetened juices, carbonated soft drinks (like Coca-Cola), ice cream, biscuits and confectionary.

New Brazilian Dietary Guidelines

In 2014, the Brazilian government released its new and unique nutritional advice to its people. While other countries persisted with their food pyramid, and their populations continued to ignore their advice, Brazil published its NOVA food classification. It advised people to:

- Avoid ultra-processed foods (NOVA 4)
- Avoid snacking between meals
- Make time for wholesome foods
- Eat regular meals and eat in company if possible
- Learn how to cook if they could not cook already
- Be wary of all forms of food advertising

There was, as might be expected, a strong response to the NOVA system from the food industry, who were keen to preserve belief that all food is processed in some way. A series of scientific articles (which had not undergone the normal peer-review process) criticized the new guidelines, but it transpired that these articles were written by scientists employed by the food industry and therefore were biased.

The NOVA food classification is now globally recognized and I am sure will eventually replace the food pyramids, or the more recent MyPlate/Eatwell plate guidance from American and British nutritionists. Although the current US and UK guidelines seem sensible, they ignore the fact that most of the food that they recommend is not being eaten, in favour of tastier, cheaper and more convenient ultra-processed types of food.

Since the NOVA guidelines were released by the Brazilian government, several neighbouring South American countries have expressed concern that ultra-processed foods were harming their populations, with rising obesity and diabetes rates. Now Peru, Ecuador and Uruguay have asked people to avoid ultra-processed food in the hope of reversing their growing health crises.

The benefit of the classification of foods into either ultra-processed or not ultra-processed is that the effects of these foods can finally be measured. Large studies from Brazil, the US, Spain and France have proven, once and for all, our suspicion that ultra-processed foods cause obesity. Further studies have implicated modern foods in a whole range of other modern diseases, as we expected, from heart disease to depression to stomach upsets. A recent study from France, which analysed the eating habits of 100,000 people, found a troubling link between ultra-processed foods and cancer. A 2019 British study looking into the eating habits of over 19,000 participants found that each portion of processed foods consumed per day increased your annual risk of dying by 18 per cent.

Now that UPFs can be classified, we can expect to see many more studies linking them to obesity and ill health. Most people get over half of their calories from this type of food, so we should probably be more familiar with what they contain. In the next chapter, we will find out exactly what they are made of, and how each of the ingredients affects our bodies – and our wellbeing.

CHAPTER 3

The Ultras

What Is Inside Ultra-Processed Foods and How Do They Affect Our Health?

We learned in chapter 2 that ultra-processed foods (UPFs) are specifically designed to trigger our pleasure-centres. They look colourful and have pleasant combinations of flavours and mouthfeel, and as a consequence of this, we tend to buy and eat more of them than we perhaps plan to. But what specifically is it about these foods that causes ill health? Once we have this knowledge, we'll be far better equipped and informed to make the switch to a healthier diet.

Let's break them up into their common parts, as most UPFs have the following combinations . . .

The Energy Part

This comprises the bulk of the food. Basic additives include highly refined flours (including corn, wheat and starch), sugar*

---

* On food labels, sugar can be also described as: amasake, apple sugar, banana sugar, barley malt, beet sugar, black strap molasses, buttered syrup, cane juice crystals, caramel, carbitol, carob sugar, corn syrup, date sugar, diastase, diastatic malt, ethyl maltol, fructose, fruit juice (and fruit juice

and vegetable oils (commonly corn, palm, cottonseed, saf-flower, rapeseed and sunflower). Originally these items would have been used in the kitchen as cooking ingredients (Group 2 in the NOVA classification system), to help make natural foods cook better and improve their taste. In UPFs they become the *main* ingredient of the food. These ingredients are full of cal-ories, and calorie density is very important in the human hedonic food code, so we naturally prefer this type of food. The amount of calories contained in a food is important in us choosing one type of food over another, but in the case of UPFs the danger comes from the other ingredients packaged up with these cal-ories. As we will learn in chapter 4, sugar, refined carbs and vegetable oils all interfere with insulin signalling and disrupt our normal ability to control our weight subconsciously.

Emulsifiers

Fat and water don't mix naturally, so foods that have a com-bination of fat-soluble and water-soluble ingredients need something that will mix them together, which is where emulsi-fiers come in. Emulsifiers have one part that attracts water (and anything that is mostly water) and one part that attracts oil. When they are added to foods and sauces that contain oil and water, and those foods are whisked up so that the globules of oil are broken down, the emulsifier works to bind the oil and water parts together so that they don't separate. Chefs use

---

concentrate), galactose, glucose solids, grape sugar, high-fructose corn syrup, honey, invert sugar, lactose, locust bean gum, maltodextrin, maltose, mannose, molasses, panocha, refiners syrup, rice syrup, sorbitol, sucrose, treacle, turbinado sugar and xanthan gum.

natural emulsifiers such as egg yolk, mustard and honey to bind delicious sauces such as hollandaise, dijonnaise and salad vinaigrette.

Common UPFs that need an emulsifier include any food in the baking section of the supermarket, as well as cottage cheese, ice cream, almond and soy milk, creams, condiments and sauces. The problem with the emulsifiers used in UPFs is that they are not natural foods; they are man-made chemicals. The main ones to be aware of are polysorbate 80 (E433) and carboxymethyl cellulose (E466), as these have been implicated in the development of metabolic syndrome (obesity and diabetes) and can disrupt the lining of the intestine (just as they are designed to disrupt the foods they are found in), causing inflammation, colitis and immune problems.

Preservatives

As described in the previous chapter, these are essential to prolong the shelf life of UPFs by delaying bacterial or fungal overgrowth – examples include calcium propionate, sodium nitrates and sulphites (which have been implicated in bowel upsets, rashes, ADHD, autism, colon cancer and asthma). Others are used to stop food going rancid due to oxidation – examples include butylated hydroxyanisole and hydroxytoluene (which carry a potential cancer risk).

Anti-Caking Agents

Have you ever visited a restaurant in a tropical, humid country and noticed rice grains in the salt shaker? The rice is a great example of a natural anti-caking agent. It acts to stop the salt absorbing moisture from the atmosphere and clumping together. The rice grains do their job by attracting moisture more strongly than salt, keeping the salt dry and in powder form.

In processed foods, anti-caking agents are needed to stop flours and powders clumping together. Commonly used ones are sodium ferrocyanide, silicon dioxide, sodium bicarbonate, calcium silicate and tricalcium phosphate.

Why We Now Eat Trees

Wood pulp, also known as cellulose (E460),* is one of the most common ingredients in processed foods. It is made from long carbon chains (C-C-C) in plants that are indigestible by humans, and so travels straight through us!

Cellulose begins as sawdust treated with chemicals at high pressure and temperature to extract the cellulose. The beauty of cellulose as an additive in processed foods is that it acts as an emulsifier, an anti-caking agent and a 'bulking agent' or filler making food look bigger and tastier.

Sawdust, being very cheap cellulose, is regularly used in processed foods and can be found in white bread, artificial cheese, vegan meat, ice cream, crackers, pizza crust, pancake mixes, cakes, 'healthy' snack bars, chicken nuggets, many 'diet' foods, jellies, pie fillings and sauces.

Basically, just as with paper and cardboard manufacturing, most processed foods **contain wood in the form of cellulose**.

* *Cellulose on food labels, aka cellulose gum, powdered cellulose, microcrystalline cellulose, carboxymethylcellulose, and microcrystalline cellulose or MCC.*

Flavourings

In the same way that processed foods have no colour (they are grey until colour is added), they also have no flavour. But thanks to the *flavour industry*, we now have artificially produced flavours that can mimic the tastes of natural foods. These artificial flavours are synthetic chemical compounds that are not derived from any natural or edible substance. Instead, each flavour is painstakingly developed in the lab. The flavour industry creates, produces and sells its flavouring globally, and as the amount of ultra-processed foods consumed increases, so this industry will become more and more important. Not only will it produce flavours that mimic those contained in real foods, but food scientists will innovate to produce completely new flavour combinations (like tutti-frutti) that are pleasing to humans but could never be found in nature. Once developed (and patented), popular flavours can be invaluable assets to a food flavour company. The estimated worth of the food flavour industry in 2021 was $12.7 billion.

In 2018, despite apparently rigorous safety testing, six chemical flavourings were removed from the market by the US Food and Drug Administration (FDA) due to the risk of cancer development (in animal testing). These flavours – benzophenone, ethyl acrylate, eugenol methyl ether, myrcene, pulegone and pyridine – were used to imitate the natural flavours of citrus, mint, peppermint and cinnamon, and were used in cakes, candies and chewing gum. The FDA also banned the use of these flavourings in vapes.

From a human perspective, the problem with food flavourings is that sometimes they can be so authentic that they play tricks on our minds and bodies. For instance, if a vitamin or a mineral is at a low level in our bodies, we will start to crave and consume the food containing it. If your vitamin C levels are low, you will start to desire foods that taste of citrus (this is the clue that nature gives us that vitamin C is present in a food). By the same logic, you might find a processed food that has the taste of citrus and, because of the taste, overconsume it. But it won't matter how much of this food you take in, it will not provide the vitamin your body requires. In fact, as we have learned, the food or drink is likely to be lacking in any type of nutrition, and instead be packed with unhealthy types of calories (i.e. sugar, wheat and unnatural oils).

There are 1,300 food flavourings approved by the FDA in the US, but it is very difficult to identify which individual flavourings are contained in a food product. The flavour recipes are shrouded in secrecy (think of the cost to Coca-Cola if their flavour combinations were copied), so all the food company needs to do is include 'added flavourings' on the ingredient label.

Although there appears to be a paucity of research analysing the long-term effects of the consumption of flavourings on human health, we do know that they can cause the following conditions: allergies, headaches, nausea, dizziness, fatigue and DNA damage.

Protein Powders

Natural proteins from meat and vegetables can be converted to protein powder by mixing them with hydrogen chloride (the same acid that is present in our stomachs), or by adding a digestive enzyme called trypsin (which is obtained from animal pancreases, or for vegetarians from papaya or fig). These 'hydrolysed protein powders' can be sourced from milk protein (whey), animal bone, cartilage and skin (gelatin), cow skin (bovine collagen) or vegetable sources (pea, rice or hemp). They are the same protein powders that bodybuilders and other athletes use as supplements with a view to gaining muscle. Hydrolysed proteins are also used for food flavouring and in pet foods, and these artificially produced proteins make up a large proportion of the recently popular artificial 'vegan meat'. They can cause anxiety, asthma, attention deficit syndrome, bloating, diarrhoea, confusion, dizziness, drowsiness, insomnia and heart problems.

Colourings

As we learned from our food scientists, humans like their food to be brightly coloured, and prefer a variety of colours on their plates. We know that most of the natural food colourings that plants produce (with their phytochemicals) also have the added health benefits of being anti-inflammatory and antioxidant. We subconsciously know that brightly coloured fruits and vegetables are naturally healthy. If a food looks good, we think it is likely to be good for us.

Matching Colour with Flavour

The natural colour of highly processed foods can be anything from a muddy beige to light grey – highly unappetizing, particularly if you factor in the bland and chemical taste before flavourings are added. After a flavour has been added to a processed food, an appropriate colouring will often be chosen. The colour is likely to be similar to the colour of the natural foods that the flavour is trying to mimic. For instance, a lemon- or banana-flavoured food would be coloured yellow, a cherry-flavoured food or drink would be coloured red, and a mint-flavoured food would be matched with a green colour.

To change the colour of the food, two types of dyes can be used: natural food colourings, which are extracted from plants, or synthetic man-made colours that are generally derived from coal tar.

Natural Food Colourings

Natural food colourings have been used for hundreds of years. The most commonly used are:

CHLOROPHYLL

The most widespread natural pigment found on earth. It is responsible for the green colour of our rainforests and grasslands, and the algae and plankton in our lakes and oceans. The natural green colouring is used to make mint- and lime-flavoured foods, such as ice cream, appear the same colour as the natural food. Green chlorophyll dyes are oils and are commonly extracted from spinach, parsley and nettles.

CAROTENOIDS

These colourings give food a warm orange, yellow or red colour. Carotenoids are extracted from carrots, sweet potatoes, red peppers, tomatoes, saffron and pumpkin, and are used to colour soft drinks as well as artificial dairy products such as margarine and processed cheese.

CURCUMIN (TURMERIC)

This pigment imparts a deep yellow/orange colour to foods. It can be found in processed soups, pickles and sweets.

BETANIN

This pigment imparts a deep purple colour and is naturally found in and extracted from beetroot. It can be unstable and lose its colour when exposed to light, and is therefore used in limited amounts in ice cream and yogurts.

ANTHOCYANINS

This red, blue or purple pigment occurs naturally in blackcurrants, cherries, strawberries and red cabbage. The pigment's colour changes depending on the acidity of its surroundings, changing from blue towards red as the acidity increases. It is used in soft drinks, jams and confectionary.

Artificial Food Colourings

As the demand for food colouring has grown over the last few decades, so the price of natural food colourings has increased. As well as the rising cost, another disadvantage of natural food colourings for manufacturers is their instability – after a period of time, their colouring starts to fade. It is for these reasons that artificial food colourings are now more commonly used in your food. These colours are brighter, less likely to fade, heat-resistant and, importantly, much cheaper than their natural counterparts.

Most artificial food colourings originate from coal tar and are therefore not technically food. However, food companies have managed to get them passed as fit for human consumption by reassuring the food safety agencies of many countries that in small doses they are not dangerous. There is no consensus on this, however, as certain artificial food dyes are banned in some countries and not in others, and some governments have asked that selected dyes should be 'voluntarily withdrawn' by food companies.

Artificial food dyes have been strongly linked to many modern diseases including inflammatory and autoimmune conditions (asthma, arthritis, fibromyalgia, colitis), cancer risk, hyperactivity, attention deficit disorders and allergies.

It is testament to the power of the food industry in influencing government safety standard thresholds that artificial food dyes remain legal. We eat with our eyes – and without vivid food colourings, the whole edifice of the processed food industry would collapse. These foods would suddenly look bland and unpalatable. They would not sell. A lot of money is at stake.

Now we understand the various components that make up ultra-processed foods, let's look at one type of product we might not naturally assume to be ultra-processed, and yet is often marketed as both healthy and sustainable . . .

The Rise of Vegan Meat

Veganism, the avoidance of any animal-derived food, is becoming increasingly popular, particularly among younger people living in affluent Western countries. The movement has grown partly based on concerns that animals on farms are not treated humanely and are killed early and cruelly, as well as an awareness of the impact animal emissions have on global warming.*

---

* What is ignored is that the carbon emissions of a cow originate from the carbon it has eaten in the grass/hay of its diet. The cow is built from the carbon of the grass; the cow's carbon emissions originate from the grass it has eaten and will return to newly growing grass as part of the carbon cycle explained in chapter 5. Animal carbon emissions, unlike the emissions generated by burning oil or coal, are therefore carbon-neutral.

Vegans believe that it is not only cruel to eat animal products but that livestock farming also damages the environment and endangers the existence of humanity. These concerns are magnified and accentuated by the polarizing effect of social media.

Despite the recent popularity of veganism, humans are hardwired to enjoy the taste and texture of meat. It's unavoidable, it's part of the rich tapestry of our genes – a type of survival mechanism. Even the most ardent vegan, animal rights campaigner or environmentalist cannot avoid or deny these inherited food preferences; they are not a choice. Our friends in the food industry, seeing the globalist vegan trend and understanding our instinctive love of meat (they cracked the human taste code many years ago), saw an incredible opportunity for a new and hugely profitable market – vegan (or plant-based) meat.

Food scientists have now been able to successfully and accurately mimic the colour, texture and flavour of meat. These newly invented – and ultra-processed – vegan meats, made by companies such as Impossible Foods and Beyond Meat, have recently become increasingly popular, driven not only by environmental and animal cruelty concerns but also the (incorrect) perception that animal meat is bad for our health. Vegan meats are marketed cleverly as healthy (because they are not meat), clean for the environment (saving the planet) and humane (saving animals on farms from ever needing to exist). The perception of a healthy and environmentally friendly food that is tasty is gaining widespread popularity. Unilever have a global sales target for plant-based meats of $1 billion by 2025. The plant-based meat market as a whole was worth $7.9 billion in 2022, expected to grow to over $15 billion within the next five years.

But leaving aside the animal cruelty and environmental arguments for eating plant-based meats, are they actually more beneficial for our health? As part of the research for this book, and encouraged by a vegan friend, I decided to try out the new vegan meat. We ordered a vegan burger from a fast-food restaurant, and within fifteen minutes our delivery driver had arrived. The burger looked identical to a real meat burger, with the obligatory lettuce and ketchup layers. It tasted like meat, and had the same consistency and chewiness as authentic meat. It felt good as it was swallowed, and seemed as filling as you would expect. However, as I contemplated this miracle food development and my body started to digest and absorb the contents of the vegan burger, I started to feel different. We have all experienced the slight nausea, bloating and general feeling of having consumed something unhealthy after eating fast food, but this seemed to be far worse. It felt as if I was digesting something highly processed and highly artificial. As the flavours unravelled in my mouth, I experienced an unpleasant aftertaste, and the same artificial ingredients unravelled and absorbed into my body, becoming part of me, causing untold metabolic and inflammatory confusion within. The feeling I got from my vegan-meat tasting experience was that maybe this miracle food wasn't quite as healthy, or wholesome, as advertised.

What Is in Vegan Meat?

Vegan meat is made from a combination of different types of flour (potato starch, soy, wheat, pea), hydrolysed proteins, vegetable oils (usually canola and coconut), cellulose (wood pulp), colourings and flavourings. Ultra-processing removes most of the food's natural vitamins so these are added, along with iron. The taste of meat comes from the haem molecule. This is found in the haemoglobin of an animal's blood and gives meat its taste. Haem is also present in vegetables and can be chemically extracted from them, but more commonly it is harvested from genetically engineered fungus. The natural colour of plant-based meat is grey, so it is coloured with annatto (E160b), a red-orange dye. Beetroot juices are used to give the meat the illusion of bleeding when it is cut.

Plant-based meat is derived from highly refined vegetables, seed oils and trees, but it does not provide the beneficial effects of consuming vegetables. The health-giving phytochemicals in vegetables, which provide anti-inflammatory and antioxidant effects, are stripped away early in the processing. Plant-based meat substitutes are ultra-processed foods that happen to be derived from vegan base ingredients, in the same way that an Oreo is ultra-processed but also vegan-friendly. They should not be distinguished as different, as they potentially have the same damaging health effects as any other ultra-processed food, whether it be flavoured and coloured ice cream, crackers, bread, or even the addictive crisp-like snack of our modern kitchen of the future.

Rise of Western Diseases

I was recently on a transatlantic flight to the Caribbean. As we were taxiing to take off, the air steward warned us on the intercom that a child on the flight suffered from a severe *airborne* peanut allergy. The allergic reaction in this poor sufferer could be triggered even if a person across the aisle opened a pack of peanuts. Are food allergies, particularly in children, getting more common and more extreme?

We have learned in our deep dive into ultra-processed foods that they contain additives that are not foods. These additives have individually been linked to numerous conditions that have become more and more prevalent in the developed world over the last thirty to forty years, including neurological conditions such as attention deficit disorder, hyperactivity, autism and Alzheimer's. They can increase the risk of cancer (in animal tests) and contribute to inflammatory and autoimmune diseases including asthma and painful arthritis. Severe and sometimes life-threatening allergies are on the rise, particularly in young children.

The link between individual food additives and these conditions is well known. Government food safety agencies justify not banning these substances from food because, although single additives have been linked to these diseases, they are deemed acceptable to eat in low doses. However, we are consuming *multiple* and diverse types of additives within each ultra-processed food item. The effect of mixing these additives together is unknown because it is not tested. My opinion is that processed food additives are the underlying cause of many of the modern diseases affecting us today.

Somaliland

Many people will remember the terrible famine in Ethiopia in the mid-1980s that inspired Bob Geldof to organize the Live Aid charity concerts in London and the US, and the 'Do They Know It's Christmas?' benefit song. The Live Aid charity generated much-needed funds to send food and medical aid to those in need, and saved countless lives. However, the charity was not able to prevent the numerous famines that followed in the Horn of Africa, with the suffering of the populations of Sudan and Somalia exacerbated by long and ongoing civil wars.

In this area there is now an oasis of calm in a country called

Somaliland. This is a country, not yet recognized internationally, which declared its independence from Somalia (which is still riven by tribal conflict). Somaliland has its own army to protect its borders, and a government that is stable and helps its people. There have been no severe famines in this region for decades. The population remain poor and cannot afford to buy imported processed food, so they continue to grow and consume their own food, and because of this they are remarkably healthy. Even the elderly have pristine teeth with no decay (without the need for toothpaste), and heart disease, asthma and Alzheimer's are almost unknown conditions. They rarely suffer from diabetes, hypertension, fibromyalgia or inflammatory bowel conditions (IBD). Their children don't suffer from attention deficit or hyperactivity disorders. There is no epidemic of allergies.

The people of Somaliland have some protection against these diseases, as they are not (yet) exposed to the artificial additives of processed foods, and the natural foods they eat contain those plant phytochemicals that act like anti-inflammatory drugs. This remarkably healthy population, whose elders survived those earlier times of famine, remain resistant to modern diseases. While famines recede into distant memory in Somaliland, the tide of obesity and Western medical illnesses, with their own death and suffering, sweeps over much of the rest of the world.

CHAPTER 4

It's Not the Calories in the Food, It's the Food in the Calories

Explaining the Weight-Gain Signals in Food

The Primate Zoo

The summer before I started medical school, I travelled around Europe by train with a friend. One of the most vivid moments of this holiday, etched to this day in my memory, was when we visited Barcelona Zoo. It was mid-summer, and the temperature was sweltering as we walked around. I have always been fascinated by monkeys, so we headed to their enclosures first. As we neared the area housing the white-faced monkeys (the ones with the black bodies), I noticed one of them standing right up against the bars, ready to greet us. As I approached, it stared at me and held its hand outstretched, like an old beggar behind bars, as if asking me for something. In its other hand, between its thumb and fingers, it held a freshly lit cigarette. The monkey looked me deep in the eyes with the most pleading, heartbreakingly sad stare. Then it took a nonchalant drag on the cigarette and exhaled smoke through its pursed lips. The animal had cruelly been taught to smoke as a party trick and was now a nicotine addict, incarcerated for life away from its natural home. That mournful, primate-to-primate stare, deep into my eyes, is something I will never forget.

We humans share 98 per cent of our DNA with chimpanzees, our primate cousins. We are identical in many ways, sharing our core drives and desires. We both like to play and make friends, we remember and learn and mimic, we have a sense of right and wrong and occasionally we will start a war with another tribe. Chimpanzees also prefer cooked and processed foods to their normal raw diet, although they don't have the capacity to cook food as they never mastered fire. We humans think like monkeys, with primate brains; tamed by the religions and laws we created, we were able to build large and successful societies without anarchy.

Imagine that you go to a zoo, and while visiting the chimpanzee enclosure you notice that this zoo has a different way of feeding their resident monkeys. Instead of the zookeeper visiting the enclosure at the designated feeding times to give the monkeys their bananas, oranges, mangos and nuts, the monkeys have food available all the time. To access their food, all they have to do is press either a green or a red button and the chosen food will automatically appear in a delivery hatch. In this way, the zookeeper has more free time to work on other tasks. The zoo wants its animals to be happy, so they give more food choice to their chimps. When they press the green button, a variety of fresh fruits and nuts appear in the hatch, but when they press the red button a variety of human processed foods appear – in the form of cakes, chocolate bars, crackers, crisps, biscuits and sweet drinks.

You notice that the monkey enclosure is full of discarded food wrappers. The green button to give them fresh fruit has been generally ignored. The monkeys seem happy enough, sitting in their branches, snacking away on their favourite bars and screeching, grooming, fighting and playing, but in this enclosure there is a difference. Most of the monkeys are obese and some of them are carrying so much extra fat that they can't move around or climb easily.

What would you think if you visited this zoo? Would you congratulate it for treating the monkeys to delicious foods or would you report it for animal cruelty?

Now transport your mind to your local supermarket, and this time imagine inside that food enclosure the chimpanzee's bright human cousin, *Homo sapiens*, pushing trolleys of food around. Our chimp brains choose mainly sweet-tasting processed foods with brightly coloured packaging. Many of these captive humans are prone to disease and most are carrying far too much weight.

We have created our own cruel zoo, with many addictive, but perfectly legal, artificial foods available to us. But, despite our intelligence, we have also created confusion about why this food makes us sick. In the last chapter, we learned how modern, ultra-processed foods can cause inflammatory and neurological diseases and allergies, but how do these foods make us gain weight so easily? Is it really just the calories contained within them?

Foods That Signal Weight Gain

The traditional theory linking modern processed food to obesity is that these foods are packed with calories and taste delicious, so we overeat them and take in more calories than we burn, storing the excess energy as fat. But as we learned in chapter 1, weight gain and obesity are not under conscious control. If our weight anchor is stable, then we will subconsciously compensate for overeating by increasing our metabolism to burn off more energy, and decreasing our appetite to take in less. Our weight controls itself in a similar way to our hydration: if we drink too much water, the body compensates by passing more urine, we don't suddenly start retaining water.

So, why does our body not regulate its weight when we take in processed foods? Why do processed foods seem to raise our weight set-point and shift our weight anchor upwards? Let's look at three of the most common additives to our diet that scramble our brain's weight-control centre and signal to our brain to gain weight:

- SUGAR
- FRUCTOSE
- VEGETABLE OILS

Modern food contains lots of *sugar, fructose* and *vegetable oils*. Individually, each of these factors can derail our metabolism, sending a signal to our bodies to gain weight. When the signals are combined within an ultra-processed diet, they can be overwhelming and lead to that hopeless feeling many of my patients describe, of losing natural weight control.

Sugar

As we learned in chapter 1, our weight is controlled by the hormone leptin, which originates in our fat cells. The fatter we are, the more leptin is signalled to the brain, and the brain compensates for this by reducing appetite and increasing metabolism. The tug of war against weight gain is easily won. When the leptin feedback mechanism is working, any increase in our weight, and our fat stores, is recognized by the brain and is easily lost by a natural switch-down in appetite and switch-up in metabolism.

Let's repeat this because it is a crucial insight in understanding our weight: if we gain fat, then *more leptin* is produced. Leptin is sensed by the brain, and the brain understands we have more fat than needed, so it decreases our appetite and increases our metabolism, leading to the weight gain being controlled (see Figure 1, on p. 20).

However, sugar and foods containing refined carbohydrates (which have the same effect as sugar) such as wheat (bread, cakes, biscuits and pasta) can block the protective leptin feedback mechanism via the hormone insulin. The more of these types of foods that we eat, and the more often that we eat them (via our new snacking culture*), the higher our insulin response will be. Insulin is the hormone that then blocks the leptin signal (see Figure 2, on p. 22), meaning the brain can no longer sense how much fat is present in the body and therefore cannot compensate for the weight gain caused by excess calorie intake from our delicious and addictive UPFs.

Historically, humans would never have encountered foods containing so much sugar and would never have eaten these foods so regularly, so the leptin signal would always have kept on working to keep weight stable. Even in times of historic food excess, populations did not suffer with obesity as they were able to control their weight via the leptin system, just as animals in the wild don't suddenly become obese when there

---

* Snacking on food between meals was rare prior to the 1960s. It became increasingly popular after the US dietary guidelines changed people's eating patterns in the 1960s and '70s. People started to eat more carbohydrates because the guidelines stated that saturated fat was dangerous. As more carbs were consumed, so people experienced more blood sugar fluctuations between meals. Snacks were introduced by the food industry to help maintain blood sugar levels between meals. A recent study of eating habits confirmed that 97 per cent of people snack between meals.

is ample natural food available to them. However, there is an exception to this rule in some hibernating or migrating species of animals, who rapidly gain weight in response to a signal from nature. Unfortunately, this signal also works in humans, and it hides in processed food. Let me explain the second human weight-gain signal.

The Fructose Switch

A recently discovered trigger for humans to gain weight is fructose. This same trigger is responsible for many animals (and birds) suddenly and dramatically gaining a large amount of weight before hibernation or a long journey. Unfortunately, this same switch is now known to be activated in humans who consume too many processed foods containing the sweet fruit sugar fructose.

Fruit-bearing plants have an ingenious way of reproducing. They have brightly coloured sweet-tasting fruits. The vividly coloured yellow, red, orange or purple fruit signals to an animal that food energy is readily available. The animal (or human, or bird) eats the fruit and takes in the precious energy gift from the plant. In exchange, the animal will disperse the seeds of the fruit that it has eaten. With this biological deal, the plant can propagate its offspring into far-flung areas and increase its chance of surviving in the future; and in exchange for this, the animal receives the fruit's energy.

Fructose sugar constitutes much of the calorie content within the fruit, but more importantly it also carries certain instructions for the animals that ingest it. Fructose is highly sweet to animals, opening up reward pathways in the brain, causing pleasure and training the animal to repeat the activity of eating the fruit. Habits are developed (we will discuss reward and habit in detail in the second part of this book). In the future, the sight of the bright fruits triggers programmed and automatic behaviours, saving the animal the energy of having to think about its actions. Each time it eats bright, sweet fruits, these habits become more and more ingrained and the plant–animal relationship becomes stronger.

But there is another important part of the fructose message to us that has recently been discovered. We know that adult animals are good at maintaining a relatively healthy weight throughout their lives. If they eat too much one day, they will generally eat less the next day. If animals are starved and lose weight, or if they are overfed and put on weight, they will tend to drift back to their healthy weight once they are reintroduced to a normal food environment. However, some animals will suddenly gain a substantial amount of weight in a short period of time as a survival mechanism. The brown bear, before a long winter of hibernation; the squirrel before its winter torpor; and many migratory birds in preparation for a long flight. The stimulus for this massive weight gain in many species is fructose from fruit. The brown bear can gorge on 30kg (66lb) of fruit per day in the autumn and gain up to 300kg (660lb), doubling its body weight. The songbird will consume four times its weight in fruit per day before migration, increasing its body weight by 50 per cent in preparation for flight.

Before Hibernating, Animals Become Obese and Diabetic

There are certain shared traits of the phenomenal weight gain of these animals. Their increased fat is situated around their internal organs and not under their skin (this is called visceral fat), they have high levels of blood glucose (as if they were diabetic), and they have high blood pressure. In fact, the specifics of this survival weight gain resemble a condition in humans called metabolic syndrome, an affliction commonly seen in those suffering with obesity. Does this mean that these hibernating and migrating animals share a common *obesity switch* with humans? A signal from the environment to suddenly gain weight?

Professor Richard Johnson, author of the book *Nature Wants Us to Be Fat*, is convinced that the evidence for this is overwhelming, and he thinks the biological fat switch is contained in fructose. In hibernating and migratory animals, as well as in humans, Johnson has discovered the fructose package. When this package is unwrapped in the cell, it causes a depletion of its energy currency (called ATP). Once this is sensed, it is a bit like a currency run on a bank, where there is panic as people seek to get their hands on the currency before it disappears. In the animals (and us), a similar panic occurs, leading them to try to consume as many calories as possible. A voracious appetite and food-seeking behaviours develop, as do increased fat stores, high glucose levels and high blood pressure.

This is the fructose signal. For animals in the wild, this is an appropriate response in order to increase their survival chances in anticipation of a future lack of available food. However, for the human there is no impending food scarcity – only obesity, diabetes and hypertension. For the animal (or bird) and the human, the fructose switch triggers the same synchronous biological changes, but the outcome is survival for one and ill health for the other.

It is only recently that fructose sugar has entered our food supply in amounts that are so high that they can trigger the fructose weight-gain switch. In the 1950s and '60s, the price of regular sugar in the US was high because sugar cane, which needs a hot and humid climate, could not be grown in much of the country apart from the deep south. It therefore had to be imported at great cost. Corn, on the other hand, is a staple American food, growing naturally and abundantly in much of the country. It remained ultra-cheap because of generous government subsidies given to farmers who grew it.

The white starch inside a corn kernel is made up of long chains of glucose molecules. Scientists invented a process, using acid and enzymes, to break down these long chains into a shorter, more digestible sugar: dextrose, a form of glucose. However, although this could be added to food, it was not as sweet as regular sugar and therefore could not replace it.

In the 1960s, scientists from America and Japan collaborated to create a process which turned the dextrose from treated corn into fructose, the sweet-tasting sugar that is also in fruit. They were able to take a cheap staple crop and make it into a highly sweet sugar alternative. This was called high-fructose corn syrup (HFCS).

In the 1970s, HFCS started to be introduced into processed foods, making them cheaper to produce and even sweeter to taste; by the 1980s, it had replaced sugar in Coca-Cola. However, by 2000 — the peak of HFCS's popularity for food manufacturers — doctors were becoming increasingly concerned at the health consequences of consuming too much of it. Scientific evidence was building that linked HFCS in food to an increased risk of obesity, diabetes and heart disease.

We now know the reason fructose increases the chance of weight gain and diabetes. Fructose is processed differently in our bodies to other carbohydrates. When fructose enters a cell, it is metabolized to produce energy. This energy is then either stored or used up immediately. This is the normal process that all food goes through when digested, converting it into energy.

However, fructose differs from other foods, as while it is being broken down, it drains the energy-making capacity of the cell. The normal energy currency that cells use, ATP, is converted to a useless currency called AMP, which is then destroyed by the cell. The draining of the energy currency tips the cell into a low-energy state, and the cell signals this change to the weight-control centre in the brain. The response to the low-energy signal is a voracious increase in appetite and a reduction in metabolic energy expenditure. This results in more energy storage and subsequent weight gain.

The Fructose Weight-Gain Switch

In response to the health consequences of consuming HFCS, it was banned as a food additive in the UK in 2007, around forty years after it was introduced into the food system here.

However, HFCS does not differ too drastically, as far as

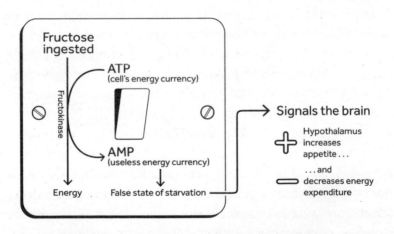

Figure 5: The fructose weight-gain switch

fructose content is concerned, to regular sugar. HFCS contains around 55 per cent fructose, whereas the sucrose molecule of sugar is a simple glucose-fructose bond, meaning sucrose contains 50 per cent fructose.

Simple sugar therefore provides the double metabolic attack of blocking the leptin-signalling pathway (via increased insulin) *plus* activating the fructose switch and providing a false sense of starvation. Which begs the question of why food safety regulators in the UK banned HFCS but left simple sugar alone?

One of the fruits containing the highest levels of fructose is the apple. This is the reason that natural apple juice tastes particularly sweet, and it is the reason that apple concentrate still appears as a 'natural' food sweetener within processed food. While the dose of fructose in fresh fruits is not enough to trigger the fructose weight-gain switch, concentrated natural fruit juices, if taken in in excess, can be a trigger to unhealthy weight gain via the fructose pathway.

So, as we've seen, by chemically manipulating simple corn, and changing it into sweet fructose, food scientists inadvertently flooded our food supply with this toxic, weight-promoting additive. But as well as being turned into fructose sugar, corn can also be turned into vegetable oil . . . the third of our common weight-gain triggers.

Vegetable Oils

We have been informed for many years that vegetable oils such as sunflower, canola and rapeseed are good for us. Often, these oils display prominent 'Heart Healthy' or 'High in Omega-6' claims on their packaging. However, the historic research suggesting that these oils protect us from heart disease has recently been proven to be untrue. In 2016, researchers at the National Institute of Health (NIH) in the US reinvestigated a famous study called the Minnesota Coronary Experiment, which was conducted between 1968 and 1973. The study recruited thousands of psychiatric patients living in mental health institutions, and split them into two groups. One of the groups continued a normal American diet containing lots of saturated fats in the form of butter, milk, cheese and meat; the other group ate similar foods but with the fat replaced with vegetable oil, in this case corn oil.*

The aim of the trial was to prove that saturated fat caused an increased risk of heart disease – a theory that was called the diet–heart hypothesis. The subjects had their cholesterol levels and heart health checked at regular intervals. The initial study findings, published in 1989, showed that the group of people who switched to vegetable oils had lower cholesterol levels, but there was no difference in heart disease between the two groups. The study concluded that this was because there was not enough time for heart disease to occur – and that further analysis of the two groups in the future would show a difference. The conclusion was that, in time, the lower cholesterol level in the vegetable-oil group would eventually translate to fewer heart attacks and longer lives. These findings influenced the US government to alter its dietary guidelines and encourage people to eat less saturated fat (butter, eggs, red meat) and to switch to cooking with vegetable oils and eating grains instead.

The long-term prediction that vegetable oils would improve health was assumed by the authors of the study. However, the

---

* A type of vegetable oil containing high levels of linoleic acid, a form of omega-6.

long-term outcome of the trial was not published by those researchers, who had set out with the specific aim of proving that saturated fat caused heart disease. The original authors decided not to publish their results when the outcome data looked like it wasn't going to prove their hypothesis. In fact, the results were effectively buried because they contradicted the diet–heart hypothesis.

Forty years later, when the NIH researchers looked at the historical data, they found the opposite of what had been assumed. Despite the cholesterol levels of the vegetable-oil group being significantly lower, this did not translate into less cardiac disease. In fact, the group that were fed the 'heart-healthy' diet died significantly earlier than the group that consumed the normal American diet. The reason that these outcomes were not published at the time goes to the heart of medical research bias: the outcome of the study did not prove what the researchers had set out to prove and therefore they decided not to publish, leaving us with a decades-long incorrect assumption that vegetable oils are heart-healthy and saturated fats are unhealthy.

This is the historical context behind those long rows of vegetable oils found in your local supermarket — the cooking oils that we as a population consider 'healthy'. The incorrect ideology that vegetable oils are heart-healthy and that saturated fats increase your risk of heart disease is ingrained in us from an early age. But the gallon upon gallon of golden oils in those rows are not the only vegetable oils present in the supermarket; they are only the visible ones. Just as much vegetable oil as can be seen in those rows of bottles is infused into the manufactured foods found on the other shelves. It is present in large volumes, but hidden from our view within tasty, processed foods.

Vegetable oils, just like high-fructose corn syrup, are made from cheap staple crops by a complex chemical heating process. In fact, food scientists are so clever that they can turn corn into sweet HFCS, or alternatively they can turn it into vegetable oil. Many of the seeds that make up vegetable oils, such as cottonseed and rapeseed, are not natural human foods, and would normally be discarded by farmers. The refining process of these oils means that farmers' garbage crops can now be sold to the oil-processing plants.

Vegetable oils are now incredibly prevalent throughout our food system, from the cooking oils in our kitchens to the processed foods in our cupboards and the fast foods we eat on the move or have delivered to our door. They are cheap to make and were considered heart-healthy until recently. But how do they really affect our health?

Essential Fats and Your Health

Nature provides us with two types of *essential oils*. We all know the mantra 'you are what you eat', and this is certainly true for these products. They are essential to us in our diet because we cannot make them within our own bodies; instead we are reliant on consuming them. They are similar in this respect to some vitamins, which have to be eaten in food otherwise we will develop a deficiency disease.

The two types of essential oils are *omega-3* and *omega-6*. These fats are found on every single one of our cell walls, and affect insulin signalling and inflammation in our bodies. In order to work together effectively, omega-3 and 6 need to be present in a healthy balance. Too much of one or the other can affect the way our bodies work and lead to ill health.

Omega-3 oils are found in the green leaves of plants and

algae in the sea, and are present in the tissue of any animal or fish that consumes these (e.g. grass-fed beef and wild sea fish). Omega-6 is present in high amounts in seeds and nuts, and the tissue of any animal that eats these (e.g. grain-fed chicken and pork). The ratio of omega-3 to omega-6 in your tissues is directly related to the amount of these oils that you have eaten.

Omega-3 has a propensity to oxidize in air, causing the food it is in to become rancid in a short period of time. By contrast, omega-6 remains relatively stable in air and does not oxidize quickly, meaning that the foods that contain it remain edible for longer. Imagine leaving a plate of fish (full of omega-3 oils) and a plate of fresh peanuts (containing omega-6) out in your kitchen for a couple of days. The fish would become rancid whereas the peanuts, containing the more stable omega-6 oil, would remain edible for much longer.

The propensity of foods containing the omega-3 oil to oxidize and 'go off' quickly means that food companies need to remove this oil from any food for it to have a reasonable shelf life. It is therefore mostly absent from all processed foods and can only be found in reasonable amounts in fresh vegetables, meat and fish.

Omega-6 oils are found in very high amounts in vegetable seed oils (the corn, sunflower, cotton and rapeseeds they are made from contain these oils). Because omega-6 oils are much more stable in air and do not oxidize easily, they are an ideal addition to processed foods that need a long shelf life. This is the reason that this type of oil now infuses the foods we eat.

The processing of modern foods means that the balance of omega-3 to omega-6 in our diet has shifted dramatically towards omega-6. This means that the ratio of these oils on our cell walls has also moved. Historically, a normal omega-3 to omega-6 ratio would have been between 1:1 and 1:4, favouring

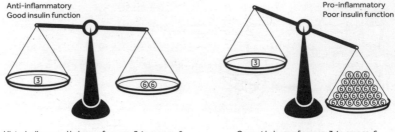

Figure 6: Historical and modern omega balance

omega-6 slightly. Recent studies of populations of people consuming a modern processed food diet have shown this ratio has moved towards between 1:20 and 1:30. High levels of linoleic acid, the omega-6 oil contained in corn oil, are now present in all tissues of our bodies.

Omega-3 and omega-6 have opposite effects on our bodies. Omega-3 damps down inflammation and promotes cellular signalling, helping insulin to function normally. Omega-6 increases inflammation in our bodies and hinders cellular signalling, meaning that insulin does not work effectively. If insulin does not work effectively, then more of it is needed to process the sugar and carbohydrates that we eat.

Junk Food = Junk Body

The high levels of omega-6 oils in the bodies of people that consume lots of vegetable oils and processed foods translate to the need for higher insulin requirements. The higher insulin levels affect the leptin messaging system in the same way that a high-sugar/carb diet does. The leptin signal that informs the brain that there are adequate fat stores fails to register, as it is

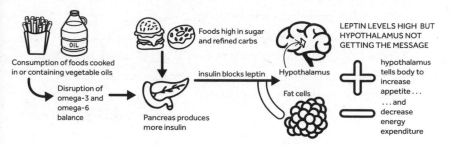

Figure 7: Uncontrolled weight gain from vegetable oils

blocked by the insulin. The brain cannot see the high leptin signal and instead interprets a low leptin level and therefore low fat storage, acting to increase appetite and decrease metabolic energy as a survival mechanism – the opposite to what it should do, and what it would do if it could read the fat signal. In short, higher levels of omega-6 derail the leptin messaging system and can therefore cause us to gain weight.

It's Not the Calories in the Food, It's the Food in the Calories

Processed food contains a lot of calories; it's tasty and addictive. But it's not the calories in the processed food that cause some people to struggle with obesity. As we have learned in this chapter, certain elements inside processed foods act on our bodies to increase our weight setting. Sugar and refined carbohydrates *plus* vegetable oils lead to an increase in our insulin levels. The insulin acts to block the signal (leptin) from our fat cells, which usually work to register our correct fat levels in the brain.

Fructose, present in HFCS, fruit sweeteners and fruit juices, acts in a different way to increase our weight setting and cause weight gain. Fructose drains the cells that process it of their energy-making capacity, and they send a false starvation signal to us, leading to an increase in appetite and weight gain.

Finally, it should be remembered that ordinary sugar, which is 50 per cent fructose, acts on *both* the leptin-blocking pathway and the fructose weight-gain pathway.

So, we have learned that it's not the calories in processed foods that cause weight gain or inflammatory diseases, it's the messages that these foods send to our bodies. These once-subtle messages originate in real, fresh foods, but when they are extracted and transferred to processed foods, they are concentrated to such high levels that they become amplified to the extreme. A biological message that might once have nudged us to a particular behaviour can now act like a sledgehammer on our metabolism, smashing through our normal regulatory mechanisms and causing addictive behaviours, the formation of bad habits, weight gain and Western inflammatory diseases.

But why do plants send signals to us in the first place, and how do both plants and animals benefit from this? In the next chapter, we will look at the importance of plant signalling to our health and wellbeing.

CHAPTER 5

Plant Medicine

'Vitality and beauty are gifts of Nature for those who live according to its laws.'

Leonardo da Vinci

London, January 2023

My procrastination was coming to an end. I had done everything I could to avoid sitting down and writing my book. My emails were up to date, and some had even been replied to in seconds; my website revamp was complete, my flat cleaned, plants watered, desk tidied, pencils sharpened, paper ready. My PA Natalie liked me like this – highly efficient (which was highly unusual). But I now needed to sit down and put all the ideas I had been gathering in my mind for this book into words. My final act before writing would be to do absolutely nothing for half an hour. Inspired by Oliver Burkeman's book *Four Thousand Weeks* (the amount of time we have on this earth if we are lucky), I was planning to savour my life for thirty minutes without distraction. No mobile phone, TV, radio or even a book.

My London flat has fantastic views over the River Thames, and I sat down in an easy chair by the window, took a breath and relaxed. The world started to come to life . . . the river tide was coming in and I became aware of the sound of rippling waves; seagulls squawked in the distance and the Uber boat droned past. It was only mid-afternoon but already the winter sun was going down over Chelsea Bridge, and the river began to glitter with golden flecks. A couple of joggers chatted happily as they ran past in their cold-weather gear, the water vapour from their breaths condensing into tiny droplets of water and ice crystals as it hit the cold air.

Catching the Rays – How Our Calories Are Made

I got up to examine Vivien, my very large house plant. She had been with me for years and was one of those plants with a trunk that looks braided or plaited.* She had recently been severely injured in the lift as I moved her into my flat six months previously. The two-man lift could hardly fit in one man and a small tree (I was pinned into the corner of the lift by her branches in a Mr Bean-esque way). She had arrived in the flat depleted, with major branches and shoots broken, reduced to half her original size. But to look at her now, as she soaked in the sunshine, she was magnificent. She had bloomed to her previous size and then more; her foliage was tropical, with hundreds of large leaves and sticky sap dripping from the fresh growth. She had reached the 7-foot (2.2-metre) ceiling weeks ago, and I had been regularly pruning the high leaves, removing bunch after bunch. But still she grew. The large pot she was planted in was one of those self-irrigating ones, with a reservoir of water at the bottom, then gravel and then soil. When full, the reservoir held 6 litres of water, but Vivien would get

* Money tree, or *Pachira aquatica*.

through this in a week. The puzzling thing about her growth was that it did not affect the amount of soil in the pot. She had trebled in size but it did not appear that she had used any soil for her growth. Where was Vivien's phenomenal growth coming from?

The Willow Tree Experiment

The theory that plants used soil as their food to grow originated in ancient Greek times and remained the explanation for plant growth until 1640, when it was tested by a scientist from Brussels called Jan Baptista van Helmont. He was fascinated by the conservation of mass, i.e. when something grows, where does the growth come from? And he was particularly interested in plant growth.

Over a five-year period, Helmont carried out the Willow Tree Experiment. He observed the growth of a willow tree in his garden, measured the amount of soil in its plant pot and measured the growth of the tree. At the end of the experiment the tree had gained 74kg (the weight of an average-sized man) whereas the amount of soil had only decreased by 57 grams (a quarter of a handful). He concluded that the plant had *not* grown through the nutrients in the soil, but that its increase in size had come from *water*. But we now know that this conclusion is not entirely accurate. Like Helmont's willow tree, Vivien's leaves and branches – basically her whole skeleton – are made up of row after row of *carbon atoms*.

Sometimes the row of carbon can be millions of atoms long, spiralling into rigid cellulose chains – providing the structure and support needed for the branches and leaves to exist. But water (H_2O) does not contain carbon, so Helmont's conclusion that plant growth was entirely due to water was wrong.

I sat down and contemplated my carbon-laden, leafy friend. Vivien's phenomenal growth and the carbon making up her structure had come from somewhere, but not the soil or the water in her pot . . . I thought all the way back to a distant school biology class, and remembered that plants take in carbon dioxide, so her carbon skeleton must have been extracted from thin air. Vivien's favourite food was the carbon in the atmosphere. As I breathed out, the carbon dioxide (CO_2) in my breath diffused into the room and Vivien sucked it in. Part of me became part of Vivien – what an astonishing thought.

So, her rapid growth came from the water in her pot and the CO_2 in the air (from my breath, the joggers' breaths, the jets of the planes flying overhead, the Uber boat engine . . .), and she harnessed the energy from the sun to make this growth. As waves of the sun's photons, which had left the surface of the sun eight minutes earlier, crashed into her leaves at the speed of light, they created a chemical reaction that split the CO_2 she had sucked in, into the carbon that she used to make her skeleton (and grow) and the leftover oxygen she breathed back out into the room.

But as well as growing, and making the oxygen that we all rely on to survive, plants like Vivien convert and store the sun's precious energy. Each of the millions of links that join up to form a plant's carbon skeleton store a charge of chemical energy. And when the carbon links are split, a crack of that energy is released (imagine pulling a miniature Christmas cracker). This is where all the biological energy on earth comes from, and all our calories (even the ones in UPFs) originate from this.

It is important to be aware of this natural interaction between plants and animals. The carbon cycle, that flow of

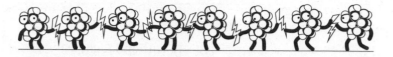

Figure 8: Carbohydrate energy train
The chains of carbon in plants contain stored energy from the
sun. When these chains are broken, this energy is released.

carbon between us and plants, is critical for the survival of both.
Its precise mechanism is ingrained in the DNA of both species.
Equally important, and equally ingrained within us, is the natural flow of *energy* from our plant friends to us – how we
nourish ourselves. This is fundamental to our understanding
that natural foods are good for our health and modern foods
can confuse our bodies and cause disease.

How to Make Edible Energy

Vivien's leaves are indigestible to me, but if I invited a hungry
goat into my flat it would continue the process of energy
transfer from the sun, to Vivien, and then into its own body by
eating the leaves. As the goat digested, the leaf's carbon atoms
would be broken (with the help of oxygen) and precious
energy would be obtained by the goat for it to move and survive. The by-product from this reaction? The goat breathes
out CO_2 back into the room for Vivien to recycle back into her
plant skeleton.

If I sealed off my apartment so that air could not get in or
out, and brought in fifty Vivien plants (and watered them),
then both the plants and the goat would survive for years. Each
is reliant on the other for their survival.

Burning Fat

How do we lose weight? The energy that is stored in our fat comes from the same type of carbon links that plants use to store their energy. When we need to use our fat for energy, oxygen (that we breathe in) is used to break those carbon chains and release that micro-crack of energy. As the carbon links are broken, the individual carbon atoms bind with the oxygen to produce CO_2, which we breathe out. The carbon dioxide that we breathe out originates from our burned fat stores, similar to how the exhaust of our car works. Imagine losing a substantial amount of weight by starving yourself or exercising a lot. That weight of fat is lost through your breath as you exhale CO_2. Weight loss from fat stores does not come via our alimentary (digestive) excretions; it happens through our breath.

The Breath of Life

The carbon cycle is common knowledge to any biology student. Plants and animals are co-dependent upon each other for their mutual wellbeing. Plants breathe in carbon and harvest the sun's energy, storing it within their carbon chains, and breathe out oxygen. In turn, animals use that plant food energy and produce the carbon dioxide that plants need to continue their growth.*

---

* Every day we make and exhale 1kg of carbon dioxide. When that's broken down, it makes 200g of carbon emissions per day. That's 73kg of carbon per year, enough to make any climate change activist who is thinking of having a large family think twice. However, our plant friends love a high-carbon atmosphere. To them it just means more carbon food is available, and they

But plant–animal relationships are much more complex than simple carbon and energy transfer – they go back millions of years. Animals are directed to certain behaviours because of the messages contained within plant food; in return, plants (who cannot roam the earth) use animals, especially birds and bees, to propagate and disseminate their species to far-flung parts of the world, aiding their survival. An example of this is the fructose message that we discussed in the previous chapter.

Food signals come in the form of chemicals that surround the calories in food. They give us information on what is happening out there in the world and guide our bodies in how to use the calories – whether they should be stored or used up. Just as a change in the weather environment will make us sweat when the sun comes out, or shiver when it gets cold, so the energy in the different foods we eat comes with signals about our current environment – signals that our bodies sense, and then react to.

Plants' Chemical Messages to Us

As well as the essential vitamins and omega fats described previously, plants also contain thousands of bioactive* ingredients that make up the bulk of the plant–human messaging system. These newly discovered plant chemicals, called *phytochemicals*, remain poorly understood, just as vitamins and omega fats

---

will eat more and grow faster. As the planet's carbon levels increase, so our plants (and algae) grow faster. Without this global self-regulator our climate crisis would be much worse.

* *Bioactive* means causing a biological response. Anything that causes a change to us physically or mentally.

were before them. Phytochemicals have many uses for plants, and when consumed by humans they trigger biological responses that affect our health, and often our weight, profoundly. There are thought to be anywhere between 50,000 to 5 million phytochemicals in existence, but the actions of most are still uncertain. Some are used as well-known pharmaceutical or recreational drugs (aspirin, morphine, caffeine, tobacco). We know that many tribes living in rainforests use plants as a local pharmacy, extracting remedies from their leaves, flowers and bark in response to an illness.

Oxygen, Oxidative Stress and Antioxidants

The earth's atmosphere is made up of 20 per cent oxygen. It engulfs us. As we have seen in this chapter, oxygen is made by plants as a by-product of their growth and is vital for animal and human survival; without it we could not break the carbon links in food and release their life-giving energy. However, there is a downside to oxygen. It acts like a biological paint-stripper, snatching electrons from anything that it comes into contact with, in the process causing cellular damage. This is called *oxidative stress*. In humans (and plants), oxidative stress causes cell death, increases risk of cancer and leads to ageing.

Oxidation is the process responsible for food 'going off' and becoming rancid. It causes corrosion and rusting of metal. *Antioxidants* are responsible for adding a new fresh coat (of electrons) to restore tissues to normal. By reversing oxidative stress, they replenish and refresh our cells and our health.

Phytochemicals have an array of uses for plants, and as a by-product some of these can also be beneficial to humans. These include:

ANTIOXIDANT EFFECT

Plants make oxygen, and therefore (even more so than humans) need to deal with the consequences of oxidative stress, which if left unchecked would irreparably damage them. Plants counteract this potential danger by producing lots of antioxidants. These health-giving chemicals attract and mop up the oxidative stress (the electrons are called free radicals), and restore health to the plant. When humans eat plants, their antioxidant molecules continue to work inside our bodies to deal with our own oxidative stress, and restore our health. Left unchecked, oxidative stress causes many types of modern diseases from Alzheimer's to diabetes. All plants and fruits contain antioxidants, but those containing particularly high levels of these health-giving natural chemicals include blueberries, strawberries, raspberries, red cabbage, beans, beets, leafy green vegetables, garlic and turmeric.

ANTI-INFLAMMATORY EFFECT

In response to attacks by insects, bacteria, viruses and herbivores, plants produce thousands of different anti-inflammatory chemicals. These chemicals are toxic to the animals who consume large quantities of the plant but can be beneficial in small doses. Just as with plant antioxidants, when we eat plants containing anti-inflammatory phytochemicals they continue working inside our bodies to dampen down the chronic inflammation produced by natural ageing and many modern diseases. Foods containing large quantities of these include avocados, broccoli, blueberries, turmeric, cherries, oranges, tomatoes and grapes. Non-plant foods that contain these properties include dark chocolate, red wine, green tea and fatty fish.

FLAVOURS, COLOURS AND SMELLS

In opposition to plant toxins, which protect the plant from being eaten, many phytochemicals have evolved to attract animals to eat them. These natural chemicals impart pleasant flavours and aromas to a fruit and give them an attractive bright colour, signalling 'eat me'. Bright-coloured fruits and vegetables also tend to contain high levels of antioxidant and anti-inflammatory properties.

The Wilder the Better

Plants produce many of their protective phytochemicals in response to harsh conditions, or in response to attack. Conditions in the wild are much more uncertain and dangerous for plants than those grown in the controlled environment of the farm, where pesticides, fencing and irrigation protect them and encourage them to grow safely. Farmed vegetables therefore contain *less* protective and health-giving natural chemicals. You may notice that vegetables that originate from more traditional farms smell more natural than those from large industrial food producers. In addition, phytochemicals are degraded and destroyed by any type of food processing, so the more the food is processed, the weaker the health-giving effect of the final product.

Natural foods contain valuable information about the environment around us as well as nourishing us. Our newly discovered plant phytochemicals switch on and off metabolic pathways and generally have a positive health effect on us.

They reduce and soothe chronic modern inflammatory and degenerative diseases, and reduce cancer growth by detoxing cells. They also slow ageing by their antioxidant effect.

The Perils of Switching from Fresh to Processed Foods

A reminder that when we consume too much processed food, we experience a double blow to our health and wellbeing. The more UPFs we eat, the fewer natural plant and animal foods we ingest, missing out on key benefits including the phyto-chemicals discussed above. Not only are we taking in damaging inflammatory chemicals and weight-gain messages from UPFs, but we also miss out on the naturally protective effect that fresh foods give us.

CHAPTER 6

On Exercise

'The purpose of training is to tighten up the slack, toughen the body, and polish the spirit.'

Morihei Ueshiba

I recently took a trip to Costa Rica with my two teenage daughters. I had enrolled us on a cycling holiday, despite us not being active cyclists. The holiday company stated that 'weekend cyclists' would be fit enough to enjoy the exertions of the holiday. Naively, I had decided that maybe just being able to ride bikes, and being moderately active, might be enough for us to savour the beautiful tropical country. But when we arrived at the small hotel, and met the other cyclists, alarm bells began to ring with my suspicious daughters, who I had assured would be enjoying the odd leisurely bike ride and nothing more.

Even at breakfast, many of our fellow guests were sporting lycra cycling outfits, but the really worrying thing was that several had brought their own racing saddles and others had even brought their own clipped-in pedals. As we ate our breakfast of delicious fresh fruit and drank our Costa Rican coffee, the friendly local guide took us through the ten-day itinerary – usually a morning ride and then an afternoon ride of around 20–30km . . . each. In unison, my daughters turned to me accusingly. 'Dad, you brought us on a BOOT CAMP!!'

The interesting thing about this holiday was the effect that quite vigorous daily exertion, combined with lots of fresh and well-prepared, non-processed, local foods, had on our bodies. We had expected to get fitter and lose some weight, but in practice we got fit and all *gained* weight. I had noticed before the start, as we were getting to know the other cyclists in the group, that many of the men, who were keen long-distance cyclists and clearly quite fit, carried a definite paunch of fat stored around their abdomen. It seemed to me that maybe exercise in itself did not inevitably lead to weight loss.

How Does Exercise Affect Our Metabolism?

We know from studies that people who try to lose weight by exercising to government recommendations (150 mins/week) without changing what they eat will only lose around 2kg over the course of a year. But we can also observe that the gym industry is thriving, most gyms are busy and there is a proliferation of new gyms opening. Things that work become popular, so there must be something positive in regular vigorous exercise.

Certainly, *stopping* regular training seems to lead to weight gain. I have seen many patients in my clinic who are retired competitive athletes, particularly ex-swimmers. They describe putting on a considerable amount of weight once they are injured and unable to train or have decided to retire from competition. Once the weight goes on, they find it difficult to shift that weight.

So, what is the importance of exercise in weight regulation? Is it more, or less, important than a healthy diet? What type of exercise might be best?

If we go back to our 'energy in versus energy out' equation for weight loss (or gain), it seems logical that expending energy

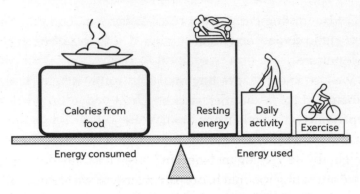

Figure 9: Normal daily energy balance
When we are weight stable, the energy that we take in (in calories) is balanced by our resting energy expenditure (70 per cent) + passive energy expenditure from daily activities (25 per cent) + active energy from exertion (less than 5 per cent).

by moving more leads to weight loss in the long term. On the other hand, moving less and sitting on the couch all day would logically result in weight gain. But we learned in chapter 1 that only a small amount of the total energy that we use up every day comes from vigorous activity – probably less than 5 per cent for most non-gym-goers. Most of the energy used by our bodies comes before we even move: 70 per cent of our total energy budget is accounted for by our basal metabolic rate (BMR).* The remaining 25 per cent of energy is used for

---

* BMR energy use is due to the energy of the heart pumping blood around the body, the energy of breathing to oxygenate that blood, the energy of cellular growth and repair, digestion, the immune response, inflammation and, most importantly, thinking. The brain uses 20 per cent of our total energy budget in BMR.

everyday movement, such as walking to the office, doing household chores, or a hobby. This is called our passive energy expenditure.

We also know that resting metabolism (BMR) can be quite dynamic. Like a dimmer switch, it can move up or down depending on whether our brain is trying to stop us *gaining* weight (in which case metabolism increases) or stop us *losing* weight (by decreasing metabolism). It can basically ship energy if we are eating too much, or spare energy if we are not eating enough. Those of you old enough to remember the Ready Brek adverts on TV in the 1980s will recollect the orange luminescent glow around the children who had eaten their breakfast porridge. This is a good way of imagining our resting metabolism – a constant internal glow keeping the vital functions of our bodies running smoothly, but capable of being bright or dim. As we learned in chapter 1, the difference in resting energy between people of the same weight, height and age can be as much as 700kcal, and this is the same as the energy expended in a 10k run or an hour long mixed gym workout.

What happens to our resting metabolism when we exercise? Does it change in response to exercise just as we know it does in response to overeating or starvation? To try to answer this question Herman Pontzer, an American anthropologist and metabolic researcher, conducted a famous experiment that compared the energy expenditure of African hunters to office workers in London and New York.

Using the simple 'energy in versus energy out' equation, we would expect that the African hunters, who averaged 19,000 steps per day, would have used up much more energy than the office-based workers. However, the study showed that the energy expenditure in both groups was the *same*. Other similar studies have shown the same results. There was no difference

Measuring Energy – Human Exhaust

Our energy comes from the breakdown of carbon bonds (as described in chapter 5) in our sugar and fat stores. The carbon from those bonds is then breathed out into the air in the form of carbon dioxide. Our breath is like the exhaust system of our cars, expelling the leftover carbon from the fuel we use. This is why when we need to break the carbon bonds faster, to access more carbon energy during exertion, we breath more heavily as our human exhaust expels the toxic carbon from our bodies. The CO_2 that we breathe out is used by researchers to tell them exactly how much energy we are using.

in energy expenditure when comparing female agricultural workers in Nigeria to office-based women in Chicago, for example, and no difference between Amazonian farmers and members of the same tribe who had moved to city-based sedentary jobs.

If the African hunters are walking nearly 20,000 steps per day, they must be using around 600kcal per day more energy in movement than the office workers.* To have the same energy expenditure, they must have adapted to regular activity by saving energy elsewhere. The energy-saving comes from a decrease in both their resting metabolism and their passive energy expenditure. A natural compensatory decrease in resting metabolism occurs as the body shuts down non-vital

---

* Humans are very efficient at walking. One thousand steps will only use up 30–40kcal of energy, the equivalent of a single square of chocolate.

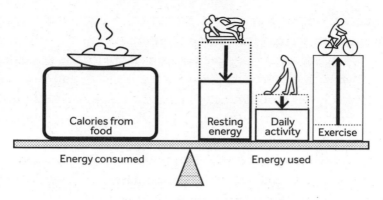

Figure 10: Increased exercise balance
The change in energy balance when more energy is used up in
exercise and is not compensated for by eating more. Decreased
resting metabolism and decreased passive movement compensates for the increased energy used in vigorous exercise. This
decreases weight loss.

functions, and the decrease in daily activity would come
about through natural tiredness. The hunters would perform
less activity than normal as they rested, and would sleep for
longer.

A study that analysed the energy expenditure in a group of
ultramarathon runners showed similar adaptation of energy
balance. The 2015 Race Across USA involved athletes running
from California to Maryland, a distance of 3,080 miles. Contest-
ants completed the equivalent of a marathon per day, with one
day per week of rest. The race took 120 days. Researchers noted
that, as expected, when the athletes started the race, their total
energy expenditure increased by the amount of energy required
to run 26 miles. However, after only one week they saw a
600kcal per day drop in the total energy expenditure (a similar

energy saving to that seen in the African hunters), as resting metabolism and passive activity dropped.

The saving in resting metabolism (BMR) occurs via the parasympathetic nervous system; the athletes and hunters exhibit a lower blood pressure, lower heart rate and less heat loss, and they feel colder. In addition, energy is spared in immune protection, growth and repair.

The decrease in daily activity (passive energy expenditure) comes about through natural tiredness. Just as with the African hunters, in the evenings the runners perform less activity than normal as they rest, and they sleep for longer.

These studies confirm that exercise is taken into account when our bodies are trying to maintain a particular weight. The more you exercise, the more your body seems to compensate for this by making savings in your normal day-to-day energy expenditure. The adaptation seems to hit a ceiling of 600kcal per day – the equivalent to an hour in the gym or an aerobics class, or an hour of cycling.

Working Up an Appetite

We know that as exercise increases, so appetite increases in response, as the body signals the need for more calories. When plentiful food is available (this was not the case for the African hunters), exercise energy expenditure is compensated for by consuming more energy-dense foods. This was the case for the ultramarathon runners, as each day the energy-saving from dimming their metabolism and resting was only enough to cover a quarter of the marathon distance. The rest of the energy required to run the race came from extra calories consumed.

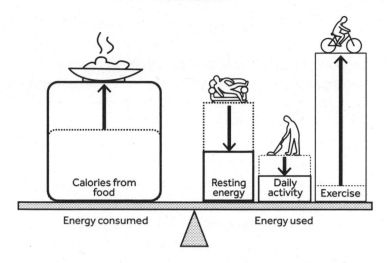

Figure 11: Adaptation to extreme exercise

Running a marathon needs around 2,400kcal of energy. For those athletes who have trained, a quarter of this energy (600kcal) comes from increased metabolic efficiency (by decreasing resting metabolism and daily activity), and the remaining calories are taken from food in response to an increased appetite.

Active gym-goers will see the same effect in response to regular vigorous activity. They will notice an increase in their appetite as their body instructs them to refuel, and they will also feel tired and want to move less, and sleep more, as they save energy in daily activity. In addition, their blood pressure and heart rate will decrease as their metabolism slows down. Just like when you try to lose weight by dieting, the body fights back on two fronts: increasing energy through heightened appetite, and saving energy by lowering the metabolism.

Burnout

In the same way that our bodies can adapt to a low-calorie diet by shifting metabolism downwards, so it seems that we can become metabolically much more efficient when we start regular workouts. Most high-performing athletes are fully aware that pushing their training too far can lead to serious health issues, as the squeeze on their resting metabolism adversely affects muscular and tissue healing and immune defences. Burnout, or overtraining syndrome, leads to muscular soreness, frequent injuries and overwhelming viral or bacterial infections.

How Much Exercise Is Needed to Lose Weight?

It seems that the more we exercise, the more metabolically efficient we become and the hungrier we get. Our bodies compensate for more calories used up by turning down our metabolic dimmer switch and activating hunger. It also seems that the metabolic saving is set at a maximum of around 600kcal per day. So how do gym-goers lose weight or keep weight off, if calories are regulated so tightly by our bodies?

As we learned in chapter 1, sustained weight loss only comes about by changing our individual weight set-point. We learned that high insulin levels in our bodies block the signals to our brain (via leptin) that tell it how much weight we are carrying. The brain gets confused with the signalling malfunction (not being able to see how fat we are), and pushes our weight up in response to too much insulin. If we avoid food that causes high insulin levels (sugar, refined carbs, vegetable oils and processed foods) the leptin signal gets through, the brain is able to sense excess fat and weight loss is seamless.

Weight loss produced by exercise works on the set-point in a similar way. Exercise causes insulin to become more efficient, meaning that less of it is needed, and this leads to the weight set-point being reduced and weight loss follows. In addition, working out decreases the stress hormone cortisol. Cortisol normally causes heightened appetite and high glucose and then insulin levels. The indirect effect of reducing cortisol through exercise is therefore reduced insulin, and weight loss follows.

But moderate exercise isn't enough for significant weight loss. Exercising 150 minutes per week – the equivalent of a thirty-minute workout five days per week – only leads to a 2kg weight loss over a year. The American College of Sports Medicine recognizes the difficulties of exercise-induced weight loss. They recommend the following:

- To maintain weight or improve health: 150 mins/week
- To stop weight gain: 200 mins/week
- To lose significant weight: 300–420 mins/week
- To prevent weight regain after dietary weight loss: 300 mins/week

Our bodies' tight control of calories during exercise (due to metabolic efficiency and appetite) mean that to lose a significant amount of weight, you would need to be active for an hour per day, every day. As you become fitter and fitter, your ability to perform more exercise in this period means fantastically low insulin and cortisol levels – leading to great weight loss. However, it's difficult for most people to find the time in their days for this amount of exercise, and in addition such extreme exercise increases the risk of muscular injury. And we know what happens when an athlete suddenly stops exercising . . . rapid and sustained weight gain.

What Type of Exercise Is Best for Weight Loss?

High-intensity interval training (HIIT) has been shown, in numerous studies, to be better than either weight training or endurance training (running, cycling, etc.) for weight loss. HIIT started to gain popularity in gyms in the early 2000s as the benefits of this type of exercise became clearer. It requires short bursts of extremely high intensity activity followed by rest periods in between. An example would be a warm-up of 5–10 minutes followed by 30–45-second intervals of sprinting (e.g. running or cycling as fast as you possibly can) and 90 seconds of slower recovery-type activity. The aim is to exercise the muscles to such an extreme that they run short of oxygen and have to break down glucose without it. This is called *anaerobic* (without oxygen) exercise. The by-product of the breakdown of glucose without oxygen is lactic acid. In order to prevent too much build-up of lactic acid (which could cause muscle cramps), HIIT sessions should be limited to thirty minutes.

HIIT exercise increases the stress on your muscles and causes a 300–450 per cent surge in growth hormone (GH) release. Growth hormone has many beneficial effects, including increasing metabolism, improving insulin function, stimulating the immune system, building muscle, strengthening bones and even improving brain function. Growth hormone levels stay high for 24–48 hours after a HIIT session, so this type of exercise only needs to be performed two to three times per week. In addition, HIIT increases BDNF (bone-derived neurotrophic factor), which stimulates neural (brain) pathways and can lead to the production of new brain cells, protecting against brain degeneration.

As well as causing an improvement in metabolism and a greater fat loss than more conventional exercises, HIIT is very time-efficient. Effective workouts do not need to be an hour long.

10,000 *Steps per Day*

Many of my patients who are trying to lose weight use their Fitbits or Apple Watches to try to ensure that they walk 10,000 steps per day. They are convinced that this will help promote weight loss. But the fashion for walking 10,000 steps per day is not based on science; it was started by the manufacturers of an early pedometer in Japan, just prior to the 1964 Summer Olympics in Tokyo. The distance was chosen because the Japanese numerical character for this number looks like a person walking!

As we have learned, humans are very efficient walkers and only use 30–40kcal per 1,000 steps (the equivalent of a single square of chocolate). Therefore, 10,000 steps only uses 300–400kcal. We know from studies on non-HIIT exercise that the body adapts by improving metabolic efficiency by up to 600kcal per day. Our bodies easily adapt to 10,000 steps, and while walking in the outdoors is great for our mental health, general fitness and our vitamin D levels, it has little direct effect on our weight.

Calorie Restriction, Then Exercise

We know our bodies' metabolism will nosedive in response to weight loss by dieting and to vigorous regular exercise. But our metabolism has a limit to its efficiency. If, for instance, you have limited your calorie intake to 1,200kcal per day and noticed some weight loss and then the usual weight plateau, this means that your body's metabolism has adapted and has probably dropped by 600kcal per day, i.e. the same amount as you have calorie-restricted. Unfortunately, you are then stuck eating 1,200kcal per day, otherwise your weight will increase. But the good news in these circumstances is that your metabolism has probably now reached the maximum efficiency it is possible to achieve. By adding vigorous exercise for an hour per day you can increase your calorie intake to 1,800kcal (adding 600kcal for the exercise). You can eat a relatively normal calorie intake and you will not gain weight (as long as the food is of good quality). Many exercisers find this a good method of being able to eat relatively normally without regaining their lost weight.

In summary, exercise – particularly intense exercise – remains, as often quoted, 'the fountain of youth', producing many health-giving benefits. Exercise to *promote* significant weight loss needs to be performed either at extremely high intensity or for long periods of time every day. Endurance-type exercise to *maintain* weight loss is also time-consuming, but can mean a more normal calorie intake can be achieved.

Now that we have looked at the relationship between the body and nutrition, the next section of this book turns to the relationship between our brains and our modern food environment.

PART 2

Mind
How Our Brains Handle Modern Food

CHAPTER 7

Who Are You?

Understanding Unconscious Behaviour – Habits and Reward

> *'We are what we repeatedly do. Excellence, then, is not an act but a habit.'*
>
> Aristotle

If you have ever attended a football game in England, you might have heard the repetitive chant 'WHO ARE YOU?!' directed by one set of supporters towards the opposing set. It is an amusing, territorial chant, but the question itself is, in different circumstances, a fundamental one.

Have you ever thought about the question *Who are you?* Your answer might include your gender, ethnic background or nationality, perhaps your religion, your family ties or whether you are a parent. It might include your appearance or your health or disability . . . but is this the real you?

Meeting You

Imagine meeting up in a room with the childhood you, the adolescent you, the young adult you, the older adult you and the elderly you? Are these people all the same? They are all *you*, aren't they, but do they have the same identity? We know that the physical bodies of these versions of yourself will be completely different – not a single atom in one will be present in the next one. We are constantly shedding and gaining our physical essence from the environment, through what we eat, what we excrete and what we breathe out. Within a seven-year period every part of you will be replaced. But what about your identity, does that change too?

The identity of each of us – who we really are – is made up of our understanding of the world, our attitudes and our beliefs. It's our knowledge and wisdom (or lack of it). It determines how we respond to different situations that we encounter. It determines who we are in a particular moment in time, and as the world around us unfolds, so our own identity continuously changes in response. Even as you are reading this book, your identity will be shifting as you learn new ideas and concepts, altering your outlook and understanding of the world, particularly when it comes to how your food affects your body and your mind.

But is our understanding and experience of the world our whole identity? Imagine a typical and unremarkable workday morning in your adult life. You wake up from your sleep and become conscious of the world. You roll out of bed and maybe use the bathroom, you brush your teeth and take a shower, then towel yourself off and get dressed. You do your own individual hair and face routine to make yourself presentable, make a quick breakfast and get into your car. Then drive to work, park, enter your place of work, say hello to your colleagues and sit down at your desk.

Autopilot

Stop and think about this scenario. You have managed to go from waking up to sitting at your desk automatically, without the need for a single conscious thought. It's as if you are an automaton, a robot in a human body, and everything that morning seems to have happened on autopilot. The way you soaped your body in the shower and your individual method of towelling yourself dry. Your order of dressing and the way you tie your laces. Your use of the complicated controls of the car and your navigation through traffic to work. Even opening and closing the doors to your home and office. All of these actions you perform in the same way, every day. Is this your identity too?

All humans are driven, or controlled, by *basic desires*. These behaviours are passed down through the generations in our DNA; they are our genes' master survival code. But that master survival code does not stop us from living and dying. The code is our DNA's way of ensuring *it* survives. As Richard Dawkins eloquently describes in his book *The Selfish Gene*, we are expendable biological vessels. We are just a means for our DNA to jump into the next generation, and then the next . . .

The basic desires our DNA provides us are first to survive, then to grow safely into adulthood, then to find a mate, and finally to reproduce. This is the same for any organism alive on the planet – from plants, bacteria, fungi and viruses to insects, fish, birds and mammals. The fly that you might notice buzzing around your kitchen is the same as you in this respect – just a miniature biological machine designed to pass its DNA on to the next generation.

Our basic human desires control the bulk of our actions and behaviours in response to the world that we find ourselves in.

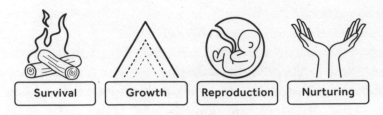

Figure 12: Fundamental needs

They are to seek safety and shelter so that we survive, to eat and to drink so that we can nourish and grow our bodies, to seek a sexual partner and to reproduce so that our DNA code is passed on, and finally to protect that offspring.

Hormonal Assistance

Our complex human machines are equipped with reminders of how we should act in order to fulfil our DNA's desires. They include hormonal signals that remind us when to eat and when to drink. These thirst and hunger signals are powerful, telling our autonomous self when to take in nourishment.

The sex hormones testosterone and oestrogen are released during adolescence, peak soon after, and then slowly fade as we grow old. These change our behaviour and personality as we age. As these hormones (which act the same as drugs) increase, young adults want to impress (for example, through experimenting with clothes) and are anxious to meet mates, and as the hormones fade these same urges begin to decrease.

To help protect us in times of danger, we also have a fear button in our nervous system that can release adrenaline. This fear reaction makes us temporarily stronger, faster and quicker thinking, to help us survive.

All these hormonal signals, which we cannot control, influence who we are and how we act; they form part of our identity and cannot be ignored. However, our biggest asset – and the most important influence on our identity – is the way we think, which is governed by our brain.

Instinctive Behaviour

We are born with 100 billion neurones within our brain, far more than we will eventually need. The baby brain has some behaviours and actions in response to the environment that come ready-wired. These instinctive behaviours, such as rooting for a nipple and suckling, help the baby to nourish itself. Crying is a form of instinctive communication to relay hunger or discomfort to the baby's carer. When a baby senses that it is falling, it will stretch out its arms and pull them together. This is the Moro reflex, designed to help it hold on to its mother.

These behaviours are natural from birth, but compared to the offspring of most animals, human babies take much longer to fully develop and learn how to survive. As the baby and then toddler touches, bites, observes, tastes, hears and smells its environment, it begins to learn. The blank canvas of 100 billion neurones is trimmed, as many of them are not used and are therefore not needed. The human baby brain is 'plastic' and can be moulded and adapted for survival in many different environments – unlike most animals' brains, which can only function in specific environments and have difficulty adapting to new ones. By the time we have reached adulthood, half of the unused neurones in our brains have disappeared.

Learning Movements

The ability to adapt and learn to survive in different environments is unique to the human brain. It is the reason we have successfully colonized all parts of the earth. Our brain is a complex machine that works by sensing what is happening in our immediate environment, processing this data to compare it to previous experiences, and choosing a response that will give the most beneficial future outcome (always bearing in mind our core desires). Our responses, in the form of actions, are slowly learned and adapted as time goes by.

Think of a skill you have learned in your life – it could be a mundane task like tying up your shoelaces or brushing your teeth, or a more complex activity such as riding a bike, driving a car, playing a sport or mastering a musical instrument. How did you learn and get better and better at doing this thing? When we start to practise a new skill, it can be difficult and require immense concentration, but with practice and constant repetition the brain will burn this activity into its circuit board. We can then do it without much effort or conscious thought. This leaves us room to concentrate on the next skill, while running the learned one on autopilot.

Imagine the brain as a thick forest. As we move from one part of the forest to another, paths start to form. Journeys that are repeated often create clearer and clearer paths through the forest. This is how the brain works – as you repeat a learned skill over and over, the neural signals directing this activity link up to create strong neural pathways. Once the skill is mastered, those pathways never go away. If we get particularly good at an activity and master it, those routes become more mature, going from footpaths to roads, and eventually becoming superhighways. If an activity is stopped, or left alone for a while, there might be some overgrowth, but the pathway will always be there, a legacy of the previously learned skill or behaviour. This is how we learn things, by basic repetition until they become automated, though despite us being able to do them we can forget *how* we do them.

The brain has multiple layers; it's like an onion in this respect. The outer layer of the brain, just below the skull, is where we make conscious decisions and work out difficult problems. Using this part of the brain can take up large amounts of energy (the brain uses 20 per cent of our total energy expenditure). This is the part of the brain that we use when we are trying to master something new, such as learning to drive. When we are learning, we have to concentrate on the new activity and cannot think of anything else. Once we have mastered the activity – say we passed our driving test and have been driving regularly for a couple of years – it is no longer controlled by the outer layer of the brain. It is now controlled by an area of the brain buried deep inside its layers, called the basal ganglia. All learned activities are controlled from this area. Thanks to this part of the brain, when we walk we don't have to concentrate on when to put one leg in front of the other or how to swing our arms. These movements come naturally and subconsciously. This saves the brain using up excess energy in learned tasks and frees up the outer layer of the brain to think about something else.

Learning Behaviours and Seeking Pleasure

But it is not just movement skills that can be burned into our brain's circuits. It is also our behaviour and our decision-making.

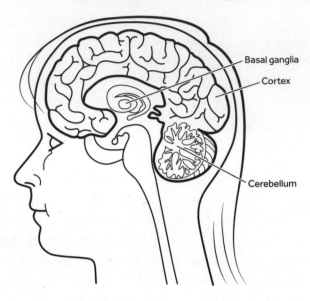

Figure 13: Basal ganglia – the habit centre
The brain has an outer layer called the cerebral cortex (controlling conscious thought and decision-making). Once an action
is mastered by repetition, it is then controlled by the basal ganglia and can be performed subconsciously. The cerebellum
contributes balance and spatial awareness (the position of our
body) to these movements.

A brain chemical called *dopamine* directs this activity by giving us
feel-good signals. Dopamine is a neurotransmitter, helping nerve
cells to communicate with each other. When we perform an
activity that contributes to our core desires (growth, safety, sex
and nurture), dopamine provides us with a flush of pleasure.
Once this pleasure signal has been sensed, the brain makes an

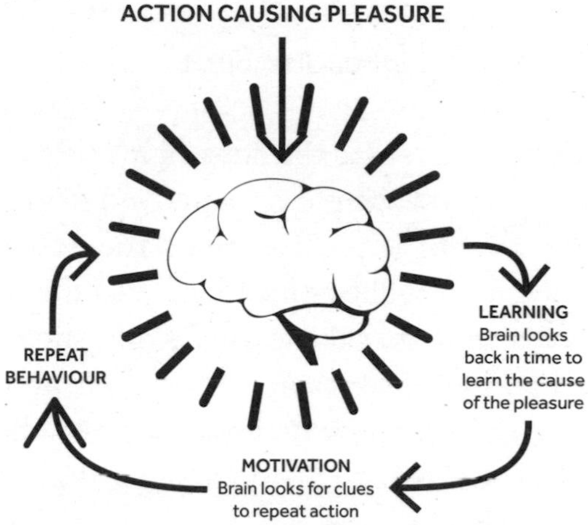

ACTION CAUSING PLEASURE

Figure 14: Learning new habits

Dopamine gives a pleasure signal, which stimulates the brain to learn what action caused it and motivates us to repeat the action.

analysis of what caused this feeling, going back in time to analyse what action was taken to achieve it. The pleasant feeling of dopamine release motivates the brain to learn how to do that action or behaviour again.

Dopamine is therefore not just a feel-good chemical, it is important in learning and motivation – without it we would have no desire to do anything. Rats who are bred to be missing dopamine don't move and don't eat. Without dopamine we probably wouldn't bother to get out of bed in the morning, but with it humanity has been relentless in its exploration and innovation. However, as we will learn, much of our modern world is now designed to trigger this feel-good response, sometimes to the detriment of our health.

Habits Are Born

Once the activity that caused the dopamine release is learned, it can be repeated, and the pleasure derived from the action reinforces the *activity loop*. The more the activity is performed, the deeper it will be embedded into the brain's new neural pathways, until just like learned skills, such as walking or driving a car, the pleasurable activity can be performed subconsciously. Once these activities are learned, they become habits – a repetitive learned activity that causes pleasure.

We should remember that our core human desires, those instructions from our DNA, are to survive, to grow, to reproduce and to nurture. Any activity that contributes to these core desires, however small or transient, causes the pleasurable release of dopamine, giving the brain the motivation to perform them. Some of the activities to fulfil these core desires are obvious – to eat food high in calories or to engage in sexual activity for instance – but most are subtle, and they will edge us slightly closer to our desires. These could include going to the gym (to increase our safety and sexual attractiveness), looking at pornography or visiting dating sites (sex), furnishing or decorating our house (safety), giving money or time to charity (nurturing), cooking (growth and survival), and even checking our popularity on social media (sex and safety). When you understand how humans are driven – what our core desires are – it's easy to see why many industries are so successful and so integral to us. Industries including insurance, medicine, law, pharmaceuticals, fitness, defence, food, charitable institutions and social media all thrive off our desires for safety, growth, reproduction and nurturing.

Dopamine Hack

Our dopamine hit does not always need to be due to an activity related to our core desires. Chemicals can hack the dopamine system too. Most illegal drugs cause a pleasurable release of dopamine. Opioids (such as morphine, fentanyl or tramadol), amphetamines (Adderall, crystal meth, speed) and cocaine trigger this feel-good response. Once our brains click onto the relationship between the drug and the heightened pleasure it gives, a habit loop can form. When the drug is stopped, the brain searches desperately for the strong dopamine signal it gave, and the only way to get this signal is to repeat the action of taking the drug. In time, these actions becomes habits. This is how addictions form. The illegal drug industry thrives on our dopamine-fuelled motivation to search for the next hit – that's why it is worth over $400 billion per year in the US alone.

The Legal Drug Store

It's not just illegal drugs that give us a dopamine boost. Legal drugs such as caffeine, tobacco, alcohol and sugar do this too, and because of this they are also big business. If you walk, or drive, down your local high street, you will notice that it is lined with shops selling you a dopamine high: coffee shops, bakeries and sandwich shops, vape joints and liquor stores. When you enter your local convenience store, you will notice that it mostly sells items that will give you that dopamine high: tobacco (smoked or vaped), caffeine, alcohol, sugar and processed foods. They are basically legal drug shops.

Eating any type of food can cause a pleasurable dopamine

surge, but foods particularly high in calories intensify this feeling. This is the reason why your local convenience store is packed with these foods and devoid of the natural foods that give you less of a high and are also more likely to perish before they are sold.

The Tantrum

When you go to your local supermarket, have you ever noticed the moment at the checkout when a young child sees the brightly coloured confectionary piled up next to it and starts pleading with their mother to buy them some sweets. The scenario plays out in two different ways – either the mother accedes to the request and the child happily clutches the sweet, or there's the alternative and much noisier scenario where the mother, knowing the dangers of sugar, says 'no' and there follows an agonizing few minutes of loud screaming and crying. If you look into the tearful infant's face (I remember this from my own children), they are devastated, hopelessly upset, shaking with disappointment.

What causes this common commotion? Remember that the baby brain is a blank canvas, carrying double the number of neurones that it will eventually need. Positive activities and experiences will be quickly burned into its developing circuit board. One of the most common of these positive experiences is the reward of sugar. It is ingrained in our (Western) culture to reward infants and young children with sweets, cookies and chocolate. These sweet treats cause dopamine release in a child's brain, and they quickly learn that the source of the pleasure is the brightly coloured sweet. As the behaviour of giving the child sweets is repeated, so the dopamine-directed learning (of the source of pleasure) and motivation (to find the pleasure again) become more ingrained in the child's brain.

Eventually, when the child sees sweets, they will start to crave the reward. They will want to take the sweet and eat it to release the rush of dopamine.

The Habit Loop

The process that the infant goes through when seeing sweets is a typical habit loop. Once the behaviour in the loop has been learned, the following mechanisms happen within the subconscious part of the brain.

To start the process, the brain must recognize the possibility of pleasure. This comes in the form of a cue or a trigger, something that the brain has learned is the ultimate source of the future pleasure. In the infant's case, this is the sight of brightly coloured sweets. Once this step is initiated, the habit loop springs into action. The brain will crave the pleasure reward and this feeling of anticipation is followed by the response – an action that is taken to obtain the reward, in this case unwrapping the sweet and eating it. Each time the reward is received, the habit loop deepens. This is the classic habit loop and it can be applied to any good or bad habit that you might subconsciously have.

Interestingly, dopamine is not just released once the reward is achieved; it also comes once the *decision* to act on the craving is made. If the mother of the screaming child in the checkout aisle gives in and places the sweet in her child's hand, the screaming will stop immediately. The decision has been made (by the mother in this case) and the reward is within the child's grasp. Even before the child unwraps the sweet it feels good because feel-good dopamine has already been released into the child's brain in anticipation of the reward to come.

You may have experienced this feeling in real life. The

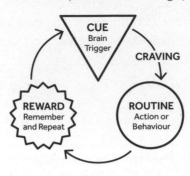

Figure 15: The habit loop

anticipation of the reward is as nice a feeling as the reward itself. Imagine you see a delicious-looking cake in a patisserie window (cue). You decide to act on the cue and go into the shop, buy the cake and take a seat. Once the cake is delivered to your table, you already feel happy – the dopamine signal has been released. You can sit there, in no rush to eat the cake, and you still feel good because you anticipate the act of eating the cake (activity) to release the reward.

The same can be seen in habitual smokers. They feel the urge to smoke – perhaps the cue was a particular time of day or seeing a fellow smoker – but upon leaving the office to go outside and smoke, many don't immediately light up. They might play around with their cigarette, have it in their mouths unlit for a while, or even put it behind their ear. All of these actions are because they are already feeling good, as dopamine has been released in anticipation of the smoking to come. When you go out to socialize you might have noticed that the feeling of having a glass of wine in your hand or a pint of beer sitting in front of you at your bar table is pleasurable in itself, even before you start to drink it.

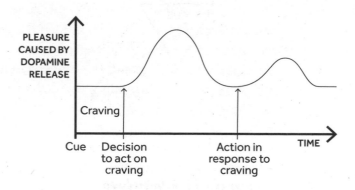

Figure 16: Pleasure timeline

Dopamine is released by the brain as soon as the decision to act has been made, giving a pleasant feeling of relief from the craving. A further wave of dopamine is released once the action to obtain the reward occurs.

Roll the Dice

This 'anticipatory' dopamine release is also the reason that gamblers gamble. By putting on a bet at the casino table or pulling the slot machine lever, they already feel good, as dopamine has been released in anticipation of winning money. The same explanation applies to people swiping on dating apps, or scrolling down their Instagram page. They are anticipating seeing something that will be pleasurable, and the mere possibility of this reward causes a dopamine release.

Each of our habits represents a small action in our lives – a decision to do one thing and not another. Habits individually are small, but if you add up the amount of time we spend on our habits it makes up 45 per cent of everything we do. These actions which we carry out in response to our surroundings (cues) make up such a large part of our current identity, even without our conscious brain needing to be engaged.

Let's repeat this point because it is critical in understanding the power that our habits have in moulding the direction of our lives, which can have long-term consequences for our happiness and health.

HABITS ARE 45 PER CENT OF OUR DAILY ACTIVITIES HABITS FORM A LARGE PART OF OUR IDENTITY

Good Habits/Bad Habits

Just as with any skill that we learn, habits form by repetition. The more we perform our habits, the more ingrained they become; eventually they become subconscious actions and our thinking brain doesn't have to get involved. This is great if your habits are healthy and good for your body. Imagine being able to jump out of bed and slip on your running shoes for a 5k run every single morning, and not even have the thought cross your mind whether to go on the run or not. The habit becomes part of you; it becomes part of your identity. But it is sometimes easier to slip into bad habits. We are surrounded by an environment where businesses have captured our need for a dopamine response. It's in these companies' interest for you to get hooked on their products, whether it be ultra-processed foods, alcohol, tobacco or social media. If a habit is causing you to move away from who you really want to be – that idealized version of yourself in your mind (chapter 9 covers this in

Why Are We Conscious?

Imagine a crowd of people walking through a city street. Most of these people are on autopilot: they know where they are going and they have mastered the complex task of walking. They may be experiencing thoughts, worries or dreams while they are travelling through the crowd, but this doesn't affect their actions. It's only when something unexpected happens that the crowd 'wakes up'. Something bad like a serious traffic accident, or something funny like a man dressed as a clown blocking their way. It's only now that they switch from habit mode and go into consciousness mode. The conscious brain is there to deal with these *unexplained situations* and interpret them as best it can, taking into account previous experiences and trying to predict the best action to take.

Another way our brain interrupts its automated processes is to settle *internal disputes*. I often find myself at the sandwich counter in the hospital convenience store, standing for long periods of time while my conscious brain calculates what each sandwich will taste like, how it will make me feel and how good (or bad) it is for me. The conscious brain acts like a neural parliament in these situations, voting and counter-voting on different scenarios until an outcome between the tuna, egg, ham salad and falafel is reached. These small decisions are sometimes the toughest of the day!

more detail) – it will affect your happiness and your health. But when we start to understand exactly how habits form, we have a greater chance of being able to change them. The first step is to identify what the habit is and look for the trigger that is causing you to do it.

Good habits include getting regular exercise, having a great bedtime routine and getting restful sleep, reading regularly, keeping on top of finances, cooking regularly, eating healthy foods, working on your relationships and keeping in touch with friends and family. These regular activities, when they become part of your life, also become part of your identity. A positive outlook on life and your appearance will follow. But it might be that your habits are not good for your health. Perhaps you don't exercise (not exercising should not be a default), go to bed too late and therefore get up late or go through the next day tired, or you rarely cook and rely on convenience foods and deliveries, snack mindlessly in the evening, and spend too much time on social media or watching TV. You might be addicted to alcohol, processed foods and sweets, drugs, social media or porn. These habits too, when performed routinely, become your identity. They are who you truly are at that moment in time.

The Future You

We have learned in this chapter that our identity – who we really are – is constantly changing. It depends on our experiences in life and our knowledge. The way we live is moulded by habits picked up during our lifetime, some beneficial and others harmful to us. But when we understand how flexible our brains are, we can use this to our advantage as we realize we are not stuck!

In the coming chapters, we will learn that the first step in changing habits is to become aware of them. What is the trigger, or cue, that starts the habitual behaviour? Is it a place, an object, a time of day, a person? What action does the habit drive you to do once it is triggered? We will learn how to develop better habits by making them more obvious and easier to perform. Once we learn how to do this, we can slowly, one step at a time, change our way of living and who we really are.

Finally, it's important to note that this change must come from within. This is a widely quoted cliché, but it is crucial to successful habit change. By reading this book you may already have learned some things that have changed your understanding of the world. You will hopefully be more aware of the effects of different types of food on your health and weight, you will understand more fully how your body can be triggered to gain weight by certain food signals, and you will be aware of how the brain's habits mould your identity. This knowledge has already changed your identity. You are already a different person from when you started to read this book, and this will make habit change easier.

CHAPTER 8

Beware of Your Surroundings
How Our Environment Makes Us Who We Are

The immediate effect of the Covid lockdowns in the UK was stunning. The government, advised by medical experts, had placed most of the population under virtual house arrest for many months. One of the only forms of escape available at the time was to put on a mask, smother your hands with alcohol gel and visit a supermarket. I personally had an 'awakening' during this time, in the vegetable aisle at my local superstore. I was in a rush, but it was a Thursday, and as 8 p.m. struck suddenly everyone stopped what they were doing and started clapping (for the nurses). I was startled and felt obliged to put down the Iceberg and Little Gem lettuces that my conscious brain's neural parliament had been debating between, and joined in with the group behaviour (I had been receiving stares). The problem was that, once we had all started, no one wanted to be the first to stop clapping, and everyone was looking judgementally at others and everyone sensed they too were being judged. It was like a scene from a zombie movie. I think I heard the clang of pots being banged together coming from the distant saucepan aisle too. After about ten minutes, hands stinging, our newly formed tribe stopped clapping and quickly disbanded into individual shoppers again. The power of the media, and the government, to change behaviour was impressive.

After the lockdowns had ended and people started to popu-late London again, I remember becoming aware of some of the changes they had caused. I observed people travelling on the underground and was convinced many of them had put a lot of weight on during their incarceration. I didn't remember seeing so many people struggling with their weight prior to lockdown, and it was worrying. I saw someone begging outside the tube station, devouring some chips with an 'I AM VERY HUNGRY' signed propped up next to him, and even he was overweight. As I passed the Nike shop, I noticed that they had replaced their normal mannequins with obese ones, wearing specially designed larger-sized sports gear. On a nearby brick wall a graf-fiti artist had emblazoned 'Thank You NHS'. There was an amazing proliferation of Deliveroo drivers. Before lockdown you would occasionally see these workers, but now they were everywhere. A gang of them congregated with their bikes and motorbikes, in their trademark light turquoise uniforms, outside the local fast-food chain, suspiciously eying the orange-emblazoned Just Eat gang loading up their addictive cargo across the road. The world had changed, and not in a good way, at least so far as our waistlines were concerned.

The pandemic had far-reaching consequences for the way most people lived. It changed the spaces they lived in and the people they interacted with. By forcing these changes, it changed many of their habits. Good habits, like going to the gym (which was banned), were replaced by bad habits like stay-ing home and eating junk. Many people cooked more, but most still relied on convenience and processed foods. Many resorted to comfort or boredom eating. People became used to the ease of ordering food delivery right to their door at the touch of a button on their smartphones. These new unhealthy eating and lifestyle habits were forged by the lockdowns. And as we now know, once a habit has been learned, it is difficult to shift, can alter your behaviour and affect your long-term health.

Many of my patients point to lockdown as a cause for their weight gain, and despite their best efforts they cannot shift that lockdown weight. Around 40 per cent of people in the UK lost some control of their weight during this time, gaining around 5–10kg (around ½ to 1½ stone). The consequences of lockdown are a fatter, more unhealthy and more unhappy population.

This all seems very depressing, but there is a silver lining. It confirms that our habits are moulded by our environment, and therefore by the same logic we know that, if we can change our surroundings, then our habits – and our health – can be changed too.

How Big Business Tries to Control Your Eating Habits

If we understand our food environment and how it shapes our habits (and therefore us), we will be at an advantage when we start to change our habits to suit who we want to be. Let's recap how the dopamine reward pathway, our brains' habits and the food industry interact.

The Food Industry's Priorities

The first point to remember is that supermarkets, processed food manufacturers and fast-food outlets (i.e. the food industry) have two things in common. They want to sell us more of the items that have a higher profit margin, and they want us to come back for these items again and again. The food industry doesn't set out to make us fat or unhealthy, but unfortunately the foods that make these companies the most money, and the ones more likely to sell, have this effect on our metabolism. Processed foods are made from cheap ingredients (sugar, flour, vegetable oils) and will not spoil as quickly as fresh foods, therefore they have a bigger profit margin.

Your Brain's Priorities

The second thing to remember is how our brains work. The brain is constantly seeking clues from our surroundings on how best to fulfil our core desires. As we learned in the previous chapter, eating food fulfils many of these basic needs. Eating any type of food will stimulate some dopamine and give us pleasure. The hungrier we are, the more pleasure we will be rewarded with. But we have also learned that foods with more sugar and oils, those with a perfect mouthfeel, will stimulate *more* dopamine release when compared to natural foods. This is why ultra-processed foods have an advantage over fresh foods when we consume them, as far as pleasure is concerned. Given the choice between an apple and a Snickers bar when we are hungry, there is usually only one winner. Food companies want us to eat more and more of their food so that our brains can begin to associate their product with pleasure.

Remember that once our brain has learned what pleasure a type of food gives us, it will look for cues, or triggers, in our environment associated with that food. When we see those signals, we start to crave the pleasure the food will give us. Internally, when we see these cues we become just like the screaming child seeing the shiny, colourful sweet wrappers in the checkout aisle. The food industry is fully aware of our immature food cravings, and will try to trigger them when possible.

Buy One Get One Free

One of the methods that supermarkets use to get us hooked on a product are two-for-one offers. The food companies have calculated that these offers don't impact future sales (i.e. even if you take advantage of the offer this week, you won't buy less in next week's shop). When more of these items are bought, more will be consumed, deepening our product–reward association. Once a product–reward association is learned by our subconscious brain, we start to crave the product when we see it or see or hear any reminder of it. Our dopamine will be released in anticipation of eating the food, and we will want to act on our cravings.

Food Advertising – Triggering the Screaming Child in You

Our world is immersed in advertising for ultra-processed foods. The adverts work on our subconscious brain and change what we eat and how we live. Again we feel like the screaming child in the checkout aisle, relentlessly bombarded with the lure of food pleasure, constantly giving in. The food companies know this, and they have learned that advertising ultra-processed foods is a great way to increase sales. In 2016 alone, over $13 billion was spent in the US on advertisements from 20,000 food, beverage and restaurant companies. Children see over 4,000 food adverts per year, and that's excluding ads on social media.

Manufacturers use colourful logos to act as a cue, triggering us to think about their products and crave them. The colours red and yellow are commonly used in logos for food

companies – red because it is associated with danger and therefore grabs our attention (think the red stop sign on a road), and
yellow because it is a bright and cheerful colour giving us feelings of happiness. Red and/or yellow are prominent in the
eye-catching logos of McDonald's, KFC, Coca-Cola, Wendy's,
Pizza Hut, Domino's and Burger King.

Fast-food companies, increasingly aware that many people
are worried that their products make them fat and unhealthy,
combat the negative perception by offering a few healthy
options to entice customers. But once the customer is inside,
when the choice between the healthy option and the tastier
ultra-processed option is weighed up, there is usually only
one winner. This applies to supermarkets too – you may
have noticed that many are emblazoned with pictures of
colourful fresh fruits and vegetables, and photogenic, healthy-
looking people shopping for them. We desire these fresh
foods and would like to be healthy and fit, but once we are
inside the store we are bombarded with the colourful wrap-
pings and healthy claims on the packets, cans and jars of
artificially tasty ultra-processed foods. Once we are through
the fruit and vegetable sections, our baby brains take over,
and it is difficult to resist food that we know will make us
feel great. If we do plan on resisting, our craving will turn
into an internal tantrum, a lack of fulfilment and feeling of
emptiness.

Even at home our immersion in ultra-processed food advertising continues, from commercials on TV to ads on social
media. Beautiful-looking, pristine photos of colourful burgers,
dripping with flavour, entice us – making us imagine what it
would feel like to eat them, starting that craving again. As we
scroll through healthy-eating ideas on social media, adverts for
fast food pop out and are consumed by our brains.

Even famous sports events such as the Olympics or the World Cup have been commandeered by food companies to entice us. Fast-food and soft-drink companies are at the forefront of sponsoring these events. As part of their brand identity, they want their product to be associated with healthy and fit people. Have you ever seen a Coca-Cola advert that doesn't show fit, happy and beautiful people drinking the real thing? Even though the reality is that some people get hopelessly hooked on sweet sugary drinks and end up looking the opposite of the people in the adverts. Famous sports stars earn vast sums of money to be associated with ultra-processed foods. Even when they are not directly paid, the sponsoring product or logo will often appear near to them.

'Drink Water!'

An amusing example of product placement gone wrong took place at the Euro 2020 football tournament. As Cristiano Ronaldo, looking incredibly fit and healthy, sat down for the press conference ahead of his team's opening match against Hungary, he was visibly distressed to see that two bottles of Coca-Cola had been placed next to him. An advocate of a healthy lifestyle, he did not want to be associated with Coke, so live on camera he took the two bottles and hid them from view, picked up a bottle of mineral water and saluted the world's press by declaring in Portuguese: '*Agua!*' This powerful statement went viral, and Coca-Cola's value fell by $4 billion that afternoon.

Imagine the positive effect if top sports stars and media personalities more regularly demonstrated healthy choices over processed foods.

The Touch of a Button

The ease with which a food you crave can be acquired is an important factor in whether you act to obtain the reward. If you are in the countryside and see an ad for fast food on the TV, you are unlikely to act on your craving if it means driving an hour into town to satisfy your desire. However, if the reward is literally within reach and requires minimal effort to obtain it, you are much more likely to act on your craving. This is the reason why food delivery companies such as Deliveroo or Just Eat sponsor popular family TV programmes or sports events. When the ad breaks arrive, they entice you to pick up your smartphone and order. Minimal effort, maximal dopamine reward – the action can be taken without the need to think.

The Food Handicap Horse Race

Foods that receive major advertising support have a huge advantage in the race for our attention and consumption. Imagine our food choices as a horse race. Usually, in a handicap race, the horses that are faster are given a heavier weight to carry, and the slower horses are given less weight. In this way, the handicapper can make the race competitive, and any horse has a chance of winning. But what if the *faster* horses had minimal weight to carry and the *slower* horses were loaded down instead? There would be no chance of the slower horses ever winning.

In a way, our food environment is like this reverse handicap race. Ultra-processed foods – equivalent to the fast horses – have been designed to give our brain a pleasure advantage over natural foods. Though we are aware that an apple is healthier to eat than a Snickers bar, we prefer to eat the Snickers. UPFs therefore have an (un)natural advantage over fresh foods. In addition, we are surrounded by logos, ads and sponsorship for UPFs. This gives the UPFs an added advantage over fresh foods when it comes to getting our attention. In the race for our food decisions, there can only be one winner.

Remember this about our food environment: our brains are being constantly manipulated by this form of race-fixing for our attention and for the profit of food companies at the expense of our health and waistlines. Can you remember the last time you saw an advert for a natural food? They hardly exist. I recall seeing an advert for a banana on the side of a bus in London many years ago; I was so shocked that I took a picture of it.

Unmasking Processed and Fast Food

Imagine a different world in which advertisements, logos and sponsorships for UPFs don't exist. Food colourings and food flavourings have finally been banned because they are deemed dangerous for human health. When you enter a supermarket, the ultra-processed foods are packaged in grey boxes and tins, with no bright colours or health claims attached. The only information available on the bland packaging is the long list of the ingredients contained within. Bright adverts for fresh and natural rather than processed foods dominate the environment, emblazoned with truthful health claims: 'contains anti-inflammatory and antioxidant phytochemicals', 'promotes long life', 'reduces cancer risk'. The bright posters depicting UPFs in the windows of McDonald's, Burger King and KFC have been replaced by grey equivalents. If you order from one of these establishments, the food – without added colours or flavourings – also looks grey and tastes oily and artificial. As you scroll social media, you are bombarded with tips on how to cook delicious natural foods, and fresh-food delivery apps promise a box of delicious natural ingredients at the touch of a button.

Picture what would happen if this world existed. Your food choices – and those of the wider population – would be immeasurably different. UPFs would no longer receive the unfair advantage they gain from advertising and hacking our brain biology. Our environment affects us powerfully, but when we see our current food environment for what it really is – purely commercial, designed to trigger our cravings at the expense of our health – we have already started to win the battle.

PART 3

Balance

How to Change Your Habits and Improve Your Health

CHAPTER 9

Change and Control

'Champions aren't made in the gyms. Champions are made from something they have deep inside them – a desire, a dream, a vision.'

Muhammad Ali

The Road to Glasgow, M1 Motorway, September 2022

My eighteen-year-old daughter and I recently undertook the longest drive we have ever done. She had gained a place at Glasgow University to study Economics and we needed to drive there (rather than go by rail or air), so that we could transport all her belongings with us. Google informed me that the journey from London would take seven hours. With typical efficiency, my daughter had me ready and in the driver's seat by 7 a.m.

We were all in a period of national mourning. Our adored Queen Elizabeth II had died earlier in the week and the radio stations were playing slow and mournful music, even the pop stations. Everything seemed strange, like the world was changing, as we sped past drab towns and cities, through the heartland of England. We suddenly had a new King and even he was sad.

The first of our several planned stops was approaching. We had been discussing our appetites and had finally decided, by mid-morning, that yes, we were both now officially hungry. The question was, what to eat?

A large roadside sign told us that the nearest services were fifteen miles away. Writ large and bright on the sign was the familiar golden arches symbol, a clever advertising man's perfectly placed ambush, preying on my vague sense of loss and growing hunger.

'I'm thinking McDonald's for breakfast,' I said.

'Dad, you can't have a McDonald's, you have to eat healthily to set a good example to people,' my daughter joked.

'But that sign was my cue,' I told her. 'Now I'm craving that breakfast. I can literally taste the McMuffin and coffee now . . . I have to act on it . . . Perhaps if I ride the crave wave, it'll go away.'

I got a sideways glance. 'Dad, that craving isn't going to go away for the whole day.'

I responded, 'Well, what if I replace the action – the action of getting an unhealthy breakfast – with one that is healthy but also gives me a reward? That's how you change behaviour long-term. That's what I'm researching for the next book.'

My daughter looked up from her Instagram feed, and rolled her eyes. 'Yeah, but what with, LOL?'

Ten minutes later, with that question still unanswered and hanging over us, we mindlessly (having been mindful of our bad food choice) consumed our McBreakfasts.

I had not considered my food choice until I saw the twin arches sign. Then I became like a robot, controlled by the beat of an advertising man's drum. Cue (twin arches), reward (food designed to taste and feel good), action (pull in and walk up to the counter). All too easy.

But how do we change the way we eat in order to cope with

cravings and triggers to eat bad foods and do unhealthy things? How can we free ourselves from these reward loops and really change our unhealthy behaviours?

I decided to consult my good friend (and new lifestyle sage) Samer about these questions. Samer, who was the Arabic translator at my clinics, had lost 50kg in weight and kept that weight off for ten years, without the need for surgery or drugs. I was due to fly to the UAE that evening, so I arranged to meet him there.

Al Ain Camel Market, United Arab Emirates, September 2022

We met in the camel market on the outskirts of Al Ain, abutting the vast Empty Quarter, as the Rub' al Khali desert is known. If you drive along the desert road from Dubai to the oasis town of Al Ain, you get an understanding of the importance of the camel in Arabic culture. Along the way you pass a camel hospital and camel racing track. The Rub' al Khali is 1,000km long and 500km wide, and in the summer the temperatures can reach 50 °C (122 °F). Before the industrial age, the only way that humans could pass through such an inhospitable place was with the help of camels. Their unique metabolism means that they can survive without water for fifteen days, as the fat in their hump is used for energy, and the by-product of this reaction (water) helps them survive. They make water from their fat.

The day was scorching as ever. The camels at the market were kept in various different enclosures by their owners. Samer pointed out the dark Emirati Hizami camels, prized for their succulent meat and health-giving milk, as well as the sleek yellow racing camels and the beautiful Saudi and Yemeni camels. He told me I could purchase one for around £500, and the thought of buying a desert ranch and having a small herd of these beautiful creatures passed fleetingly through my mind.

We had been discussing my 'fast-food' experiences on the drive to Glasgow and how best to cope with these cravings. 'You see, Dr Andrew, it is not about willpower. It is about who you really are.' He pointed to a group of Hizami camels and said, 'You would not expect these camels to be able to race fast.' Then, pointing to an enclosure housing racing camels, 'You would not expect these camels to taste good. If a man decides to lead a healthy life, this will be difficult if deep down he resents this life and misses his old one. He is trying to be what he is not. But if a man decides that he *is* a healthy man who wants to nourish and nurture his body, he will not be tempted by unhealthy choices. He will seek out good food and he will change his life so that it is easy for him to live healthily. But his mind needs to change first, then his actions will become easier and eventually his body will take on a healthy appearance, matching that of his mind. If his mind is not changed first, then inevitably his willpower will fail and he will resume bad habits.'

Samer explained that over many years he had focused on a weight-loss target but had failed repeatedly because he thought his willpower was not strong enough. 'I was like a Hizami camel trying to run fast, it just wasn't who I was. I then slowly learned that change needs to come from the inside first. Once this happens, everything that follows is easy. If I was starving and the only food available to me was a fast-food burger I would not eat it.' He turned to me and offered me one of his cigarettes (his only remaining vice). I declined his offer. 'You see, Dr Andrew, it was easy for you to turn down a cigarette because you do not smoke, you never thought to take one, you were never tempted because *you are a non-smoker*. If you had just stopped smoking, it would be different, you would be tempted, your willpower would be tested because deep down you would still be a smoker.'

Your Identity vs Your Outcome

Samer told me that trying to sustain weight loss and nurture a healthier body is like a game of chess; you have to think carefully about every move. But by understanding that change needs to come from inside first, he had finally achieved checkmate and won the game.

Typically, when we want to change things, we tend to focus on the outcome that we want. We might say we want to run a marathon or lose 2 stone (13kg) in weight. We are focused on the goal, the ultimate achievement. But this goals-first mentality postpones our happiness to a future time when we have run the marathon or lost the weight. We are trying to achieve the goal through actions that involve willpower and that we might not enjoy. The goal is reached through sacrifice.

It is much easier to achieve your goals by a shift in mentality away from the particular achievement that you are aiming for and towards a change in your identity. Instead of a goal of wanting to run a marathon, you first become the person who is likely to run a marathon. You become a runner. Once this shift in your outlook occurs, it is easy to go for your daily run because this is who you really are. The more times that you do this, the more aligned your actions (or habits) and your identity become. Eventually, you take on the body and fitness of a runner to match your identity.

In the same way, instead of a goal of losing 2 stone in weight, you concentrate on striving to be the person who could easily lose this weight. You become someone who only cooks their own food, doesn't snack and avoids processed foods. These actions that will eventually enable you to achieve your goal become easier. You find the time to cook for yourself (and maybe your family) because that is who you are. You do not particularly crave bad food or have it in the house, because that's not you.

By focusing on the identity you need in order to achieve your goals, you can enjoy the process and embrace the journey as your new habits become stronger and stronger.

To make the process easier, answer the following questions:

- What outcome do you want to achieve?
- What type of person would be able to achieve that outcome easily?
- List five small changes in your daily routine that this person would put in place.

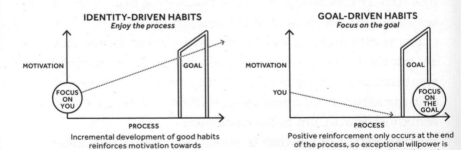

Figure 17: Identity versus goal-driven habits

Focusing on the *goal* (what you want to achieve) rather than your *identity* (who you are) means that the *process* (what you do) relies on motivation and willpower. By embracing the identity of the type of person who would achieve the outcome, the whole process becomes easier, more enjoyable and more sustainable.

Making New Habits Easier

We learned about the habit loop in chapter 7. How our brains are constantly on the lookout for what to do next to give us a dopamine reward. The start of the process is the cue or trigger – something in the environment, or a particular place or time of day, that makes our brain start to crave a reward, as it works out what to do. If the habit is strong enough, or the reward is easy enough to attain, then we will carry out the action of the response to achieve the reward.

CUE → CRAVING → RESPONSE → REWARD

We know that habits are picked up throughout our lives from our environment, our family and our friends – and it would be very fortunate if they were mostly good ones. The reality is that many of our habits are not great for us; they are just there. Habits make up 45 per cent of our actions and are therefore an important part of our identity. We also know that when our environment changes (such as during the pandemic lockdowns), our habits change too.

An awareness of how habits work and how to change them can be a powerful force for good in our lives. As we saw earlier, processed foods affect our bodies, hijack our brains' reward pathways and forge unhealthy habits. This knowledge in itself can lead to some change in our identity, via a new understanding of the food we eat. With this new understanding, habit change becomes not a chore that drains our willpower but something that our core identity desires. By changing these habits, our weight anchor will shift to a healthier place and we will lose weight seamlessly. Any inflammatory condition that we suffer from should improve. As our new habits align with our new identity, we will feel much more content in ourselves. So how do we go about habit change?

You first need to be able to identify the habit loop that causes the habit. The awareness of the cue and the response to it is crucial. If the habit is brushing your teeth in the morning, the cue to start brushing might be the sight of the toothbrush and toothpaste sitting next to the bathroom mirror as you wash. If the habit is eating fast food on the way home from work, the cue to act could come simply from the colourful advert (or sign) on the restaurant as you pass it by.

The next step is to decide whether the habit is a good one that you want to keep (and practise more), or a bad habit that you would prefer to change. A bad habit is one that does not align with, or suit, your desired identity. If by performing the habit you feel unhappy or uncomfortable, then this may be a bad habit.

In chapter 7 we learned that any type of habit will never be forgotten by our brains. If you stop performing a habit, the neural pathways may become overgrown and weaker as time goes by, but they will never disappear. The most successful way of overcoming a bad habit is to substitute a good one that aligns with your identity. To do this, you need to make the bad habit less obvious – by removing the cue – and make it more difficult to gain the reward. To stop that habit of eating fast food on the way home from work, you might alter your journey home so that you are not tempted or triggered into the bad habit as you pass the restaurant. Maybe you could assuage your hunger at that time of the day by eating a healthy snack half an hour before finishing work. Or if the bad habit is wasting too much time watching Netflix in the evening and your trigger to do this is getting home from work and immediately turning on the television, then you might make it physically more difficult to carry out this action. You could change the furniture so that the easy chair is not facing the TV, or unplug the TV and cable box so that it needs resetting, or put the remote control in a different room. This would make the process of slouching on the sofa after work and flicking on the TV more difficult. It increases the *friction* of the process.

If you want to replace bad habits with good ones, you need to make the good habits more seamless and easy to perform. There also has to be a reward in completing the action, or the habit loop will not be activated. Perhaps when you come home from work, you make it so that interesting books you want to read are handily placed for you to pick up. Maybe you put out a selection of aromatic herbal teas in your kitchen to tempt you, the cup already waiting. You could even add a small amount of honey to give you that feeling of a reward. With this simple change to your home environment, you have made a habit that doesn't align with your identity more difficult to do (changing the furniture and unplugging the TV) and a positive habit (drinking a delicious tea while reading) much more obvious and easy to carry out.

For all the habit changes that we have identified, we need to consider the following:

	Good Habit	**Bad Habit**
CUE	More obvious, easy to see	Invisible, more difficult to see
CRAVE	More attractive	Less attractive*
RESPONSE	Easy to attain	More difficult to attain
REWARD	More satisfying	Less satisfying*

* New knowledge leading to identity change makes this easier.

Let's look at another example of how changing your environment can lead to habit change. Imagine you're a runner training for a marathon. You make sure you have your weekly timetable of runs worked out and have planned your route for each run. To reduce the friction even more, you make sure that your running kit is clean and ready, laid out next to your bed for you to change into, and your running shoes are waiting for you by the door. These visual cues make the action more likely and easier to start. By having a specific time planned for the action (the cue), you will be more likely to instigate it. You might also plan your reward for after the run and have something tasty and healthy to eat and drink ready for your return. These preparations make it easier for you to complete the run. You have the cue, the time and route of your run is planned, you have decreased the friction of performing the action by preparing your kit, and you have a reward waiting.

How about that person who has decided to clean up their eating habits in order to lose 2 stone (13kg) in weight? If they have already begun to try to identify as a healthy eater, they may be much less tempted to eat processed foods and sugar. Perhaps their identity change, like Samer's, will be so strong that they have developed an aversion to this type of food. But to make bad habits even less likely, they can get rid of cues that might start their brain's hedonic craving of unhealthy foods. They could clear the house of any type of processed food. They might change their shopping routine so that they completely avoid going to the supermarket and are not tempted by the tasty colourful modern foods on offer. If they can afford it, they could instead arrange for ingredients to be delivered straight to their house (freeing up time to cook). They might want to delete the Deliveroo, Just Eat and Uber Eats apps on their phone, so that it is more difficult to order a takeaway. Once they understand why they are being bombarded by food adverts, they will become aware of the feelings these adverts are trying to generate and will know that it's just part of the world they are living in. They will become background noise.

To make their good habits more likely to stick, they could fill their house with healthy vegetables, meats, fish and dairy products. They could have healthy snacks available in the fridge in case they feel 'hangry', and make sure the fruit bowl, displaying multi-coloured fresh fruits, is prominent in their kitchen. They can plan what foods to cook and meals to prepare. All the correct spices and herbs should be readily available so that their meals taste great. If they are not too busy, and they can afford it, perhaps they can start to frequent their local butcher's or fishmonger's and get to know more about these foods and how best to cook them. They might even hand-pick their fruits and vegetables at the local market (again, if they have the time and means for this). They can plan their lunches for the week, and if they work away from home can take this food to the office.

Repetition Rather Than Intensity

Changing your character to mirror the type of person you want to become, and changing your environment to increase the friction of bad habits and decrease the friction of good habits, can lead to fantastic long-term outcomes as your new habits become your new way of life. However, sometimes getting started with a new routine can be difficult. For a new habit to form it needs *repetition*, as the more it is performed the more the neurological pathway of the action will become ingrained into your brain.

Repetition is crucial in this respect. Even if you only perform an action for five minutes, it will train your brain to expect to do this every day. The new action should not feel like it is any effort or sacrifice. It's much better to start your running training with a five-minute run every day than immediately attempt an exhausting 5k. An action which is painful or unpleasant will be more difficult to repeat.

If you are planning on going to the gym regularly, try getting up every day, getting changed into your gym gear and travelling to the gym, even if it's just to do a light workout or use the sauna or steam room. The repetition will solidify the habit of going to the gym (and finding the time to do it) and getting a reward at the end of the action. What you shouldn't do is, in reality, what often occurs. Many first days in the gym are spent in the company of your new personal trainer (no qualification required), who will take great delight in putting you through your unfit paces until you drop. The pain of the workout (and the stiffness in your body the day after) will be remembered by your brain and you will be much less motivated to repeat this experience.

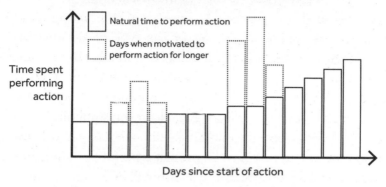

REPEATING AN ACTION, even for a short period of time every day, is more likely to result in the formation of a HABIT

Figure 18: Repetition reinforces habits

Repetition is crucial, as the decision to start an action – even if you only do the activity for five minutes – can solidify habit formation. Try not to skip a day. As the action is repeated, so the duration of the action – the time you spend doing it every day – will increase. In time, the action (whether that's going for a run, going to the gym or cooking in the evening) will not need a conscious decision to perform it. Just like cleaning your teeth, it will become part of your normal routine.

Tracking Habits

To make it more likely that you will continue to repeat a habit, it's good to have a visual reminder of how you are progressing with it. A habit tracker can motivate you to continue your good work and is a reminder of your achievements.

Traditionally, the tracker may just have been putting a tick or a cross (or a smiley face) on your wall calendar. But habit tracking is now quite popular (because it works), and so there are many habit-tracker notebooks available to purchase, as well as smartphone apps that offer tracking and feedback on your progress. You can easily make your own habit tracker in a notebook or as a spreadsheet on your computer.

Action	Nov 1	Nov 2	Nov 3	Nov 4	Nov 5	Nov 6	Nov 7	Nov 8	Nov 9
Made packed lunch	X	X	X	X		X			
Avoided snacking!	X			X	X	X			
Went for a run	X	X	X	X	X	X			
Got sufficient sleep	X	X	X	X		X			

My personal favourite for habit tracking is very visual. It's a *habit jar* that I add a marble to every time I go for a run. I had the aim of going for a run on thirty consecutive days (sometimes this was literally for five minutes) and stored thirty marbles in a mug. Every time I completed the task, I took a marble from the mug and put it in the habit jar. You can use anything to add to a habit jar: marbles, pound coins, paper clips – whatever you have to hand.

And the final advantage of habit tracking . . . the mere act of adding to the tracker, whether that's placing a cross on your calendar, colouring in a square of your notebook, or placing the marble in the habit jar, can act as a reward in itself, making the action more likely to be repeated.

How Long Does It Take to Build a
Good Habit or Break a Bad One?

Repeating an activity or action on a daily basis will eventually lead to it becoming habitual. It will be an almost subconscious part of your daily routine, usually instigated by a cue and resulting in a rewarding, pleasant feeling. But how long does it take for an action to become a habit? Research has shown that habit formation can take anywhere from twenty days to 250 days. The average time to form a habit is sixty-six days. If you perform an action for sixty-six days, there is a 50 per cent chance that it will become a habit. If you perform the action for longer than sixty-six days, the chances are greater than even. You will know when it has become a habit, because it will be something that you don't particularly have to motivate yourself or remind yourself to do.

Resisting Temptation

How about getting rid of bad habits? Well, we know that they never go away. Those reward pathways are ingrained in your brain – though as we have seen, you can replace them with healthier pathways. It has been suggested that it takes 30–60 days for the temptation to perform a bad habit to recede. You need to continue to try to avoid the cues that triggered your old habit.

In the New Testament of the Bible, there is reference to this timeframe to clear your brain of bad thoughts and temptation. Jesus spent forty days in solitude in the Judaean Desert. At the end of this time, he resisted the temptations that were offered to him.

Your Tribe

As we go through life, many of our habits are picked up from family, friends or colleagues. Humans are very good at mimicking behaviours in order to fit in with our current group, as social expectation means we feel obliged to fit in. Eventually, the group's behaviour that we're copying becomes our habit and becomes part of us.

Social environment plays a big part in habit formation. If you are aligning yourself with an improved identity and a new way of living, you will be more successful if you join or befriend a group of people who align with your identity. If an alcoholic is trying to quit alcohol, he will have to move on from the friends that he hangs around with at the bar and find a new group who are not heavy drinkers. A smoker who wants to quit will have to forsake the camaraderie of having a quick cigarette in the freezing cold outside the office with her nicotine-addicted friends. In the same way, if you find a new 'tribe' of friends whose identities align with yours – whether they be runners, gym friends or people in your local cookery class – you will be much more comfortable and likely to succeed in achieving your goals.

The Power of Now

In the distant past, our hunter-gatherer ancestors often lived in a state of semi-starvation, and the future availability of food was uncertain. Before the advent of agriculture, we never knew where our next meal was coming from. This is the reason our brains are wired to favour something that is available to us here and now over something that might be available in the future. This applies to any rewards that might help us to achieve our core instincts (to survive, grow and reproduce). Unfortunately, in our current environment of constant temptation, the way our brains are wired for instant gratification makes it difficult for most people to resist a treat that is right in front of them. The dopamine reward of eating that treat in the moment easily overrides the delayed satisfaction that might come from weight loss due to eating a healthier diet over the long term.

Immediate gratification is the default choice of our brains over delayed gratification. It is more difficult to motivate yourself to perform an action where gratification is delayed. Studying for exams is an example of this, as there is no immediate reward for the hours spent sitting at your desk. The temptation to quit studying and go out and do something immediately rewarding is strong. But a logical understanding of the long-term reward, and the formation of healthy studying habits (the more you study, the easier it becomes to study), should strengthen the willpower required to carry on.

An understanding of the ways humans are hardwired to seek instant gratification makes us more likely to recognize this behaviour. We often act like toddlers let loose in a sweet shop, their faces smeared with chocolate, their hands sticky and their mouths full of sweets. Recognize this type of infant behaviour when you are reaching out to grasp rewards that are immediately available. It's valuable to monitor these actions if they occur frequently, and start to seek more delayed gratification.

Stress and Emotional Eating

Our tendency to seek impulsive happiness is stronger if we are suffering from anxiety or are stressed. The brain doesn't like unhappy feelings and will seek out a reward much more keenly in these circumstances. Stress eating is common in the patients that come to my clinic. It is the action of eating something that will produce a reward – usually processed foods that are designed to give a large surge in pleasure. The action of eating in this case is not related to hunger, it is related to stress. During emotional eating, the body is not crying out for nutrition or energy; the brain is crying for a reward to try to reverse negative emotions. Unfortunately, the processed foods that we tend to reach for when stressed cause obesity (and ill health), and ultimately this leads to more stress, unhappiness and anxiety. The reward becomes the root cause of the problem.

Being able to deal with your own stress is a crucial tool in stopping emotional eating. If you have the ability to relax, you will be less likely to feel the need to reach for an unhealthy and damaging reward. If you know how to calm your emotions on your own, you won't have to dose yourself with external stimuli, whether they be drugs, alcohol, nicotine, sugar or processed foods. Let's have a look at some methods that can help to assuage the feelings of stress that lead to these unhealthy food choices.

A Relaxation Toolkit

There are many proven techniques that can help us switch from stress to relaxation. Some of these techniques date back to early Hindu and Buddhist teachings. They aim to calm the body, and the mind, through techniques like breathing and meditation. These techniques are designed to stimulate the part of the nervous system associated with relaxation* and close down the part associated with stress.† When you become anxious, your heart starts racing, you might notice that your breathing is fast and shallow and you start to sweat. If you practise some of these techniques regularly you will have the power to deal with stress rather than resorting to drugs or emotional eating.

Breathing

Breathing exercises are an easy-to-learn and highly effective way of switching from stress to relaxation. They act by stimulating the vagus nerve, which then switches on the relaxation part of the nervous system. We go through our whole lives breathing without being conscious of the process. But breathing in and out influences the stress levels in our system. Every time we breathe in, the stress nerves (SNS) are more active; and when we breathe out, the relaxation system (PNS – vagus nerve) is more active. By breathing in fast and out slowly, the relaxation system is triggered.

* The parasympathetic nervous system (PNS) – the 'rest and digest' part of the nervous system that is active when we are relaxing.
† The sympathetic nervous system (SNS) – the 'fight or flight' part of the nervous system that is active when we are in danger or in a stressful situation.

CYCLIC SIGHING AND PURSED-LIP BREATHING

Fill your lungs by taking in two sharp breaths through the nose. Purse your lips and breathe out slowly. Repeat this way of breathing for five minutes to stimulate your vagus nerve and feel the wave of relaxation.

BOX BREATHING

Breathe in slowly through your nose while counting
to four.
Hold the air in your lungs for a count of four.
Breathe slowly out for a count of four.
Hold your breath out for a count of four.
Repeat for five minutes.

This exercise forces you to concentrate on your breathing and can operate as a form of meditation. Focusing on an action such as breathing can lessen worrying thoughts. In addition, breathing slowly will damp down the anxiety nerves and trigger the relaxation of your body.

Like any activity, the more you practise breathing techniques, the better you will become at them. Just like with a muscle, you can strengthen vagal nerve function and will start to notice the benefits.

Chronic Stress Relief

Breathing techniques are a great way to train your body to immediately relax. Sportsmen, actors, orators, singers and meditators are fully aware of these techniques, but they are free to all of us. Once you master the art of them, you will feel much more confident in your ability to manage your

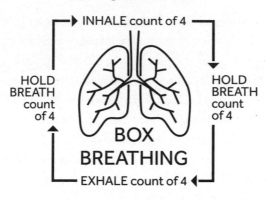

Figure 19: Box breathing

short-term stress and avoid unhealthy behaviours such as emotional eating. But what about more long-term forms of stress, and how they affect our diet and our health?

Chronic, long-term worry and anxiety leads to the stress hormone cortisol being released into your body. As we have learned, this hormone is designed to help you survive in dangerous situations. It increases blood glucose, making you feel hunger and driving you to seek out high-calorie foods that will adversely affect insulin levels, all leading to weight gain.

There are a number of activities that reduce levels of chronic stress, these include:

FASTING

We need to eat to nourish our bodies, but we do not need to eat constantly. Fasting for several hours in a day reduces stress levels. If you get into the habit of not eating (or drinking calories) for four hours before you sleep and you manage eight hours of rest, you will have fasted for twelve hours. The longer your daily fast, the better your stress levels will be.*

LIGHT EXPOSURE

There are benefits to be had from exposing yourself to light in the morning by standing outside for twenty minutes, and for a similar amount of time in the evening when the sun starts to wane. This helps to maintain a steady circadian rhythm (by training the internal clock that sets our bodily processes and hormones throughout the day).

VISUALIZATION

This can be in the form of imagining a good outcome in a particular situation (for instance, your run) or in the form of guided imagery. You close your eyes and imagine you are in a relaxing situation such as a warm beach. The more you practise this technique, the more vivid the experience becomes and you begin to feel the warmth of the sun and hear the ripple of the waves. It can become a mental holiday haven to savour, and create feelings of relaxation and calm.

PRESSURE-POINTS STIMULATION (TAPPING)

This interesting technique involves tapping, or pressing on, specific points on the head, face and upper body. These pressure points correspond to some of the so-called meridian points used in Chinese acupuncture practice. By stimulating

---

* A recent study showed that people who fast for religious reasons showed significantly lower levels of depression, stress and anxiety compared to when not fasting. The reason for this is uncertain but some scientists point towards a stabilization in the stress hormone cortisol while fasting.

these points, you create a sense of calm which can be quite pleasant.

The technique involves gently massaging or tapping on the following points using two fingers: inner eyebrow area, side of the eye, under the eye, under the nose, chin, below the inner part of your collarbone and under the arm. You often sense that you are at the correct point as it feels as if you are stimulating nerves. Lie or sit down comfortably and think about the stress you feel. Massage or tap (seven times each) the areas in the diagram below, and then repeat the process. Once you have finished, you should experience a lessening of your stress.

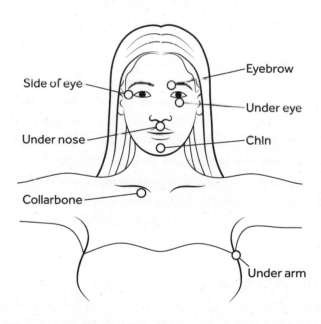

Figure 20: Pressure points

The Do-Nothing Meditation Technique

Many traditional forms of meditation ask you to try to clear the brain of any thoughts. The usual method of clearing the brain is to focus on something – this could be your breathing, an internally spoken word (or mantra), or even a black dot or candle flame (the latter is called trataka meditation). While you are sitting comfortably and focusing your thoughts in this way, the mind is naturally active yet not focused on any specific thought or concern – once you notice that your thoughts have returned, you acknowledge them and begin the focus on the breath or mantra to return to your meditation.

This type of traditional meditation is increasingly popular. However, the drawback is that it takes quite a lot of practice to be able to reach a state of relaxation that is going to benefit you. Many people try it and give up on the technique because they can't quiet the feelings of worry or concern that arise during the practice.

I find the *do-nothing* meditation technique much easier and more enjoyable than traditional meditation. You can do this anywhere, but it is best in a place where you are unlikely to be disturbed. It takes twenty minutes. Sit down in a comfortable position, switch off all distractions (smartphone, TV, music). Simply take in your surroundings in detail. Observe the room around you, listen to the different sounds, sense how your body is feeling. Sensing and being aware of your breathing can be a part of this too, but only if that's where your thoughts take you. With this technique, you are not asking yourself to stop thinking, you are simply observing and thinking about your surroundings. You will find that your mind flows with different thoughts when you are doing nothing – just observing a room. If those thoughts turn into your usual familiar worries, then return your focus back to the sights and sounds of the room.

Other Factors That Can Affect Your Levels of Stress

Sleep – Lack of sleep will increase anxiety and stress. Establish a regular sleeping pattern and aim for around 7–9 hours in bed (this will vary from person to person).

Regular exercise – Any exercise decreases the stress hormone cortisol and releases many naturally relaxing hormones.

Relationships – Maintaining connections and interactions with friends and family reduces stress.

Healthy diet – we have learned that fresh foods contain many anti-inflammatory chemicals that can help reduce stress levels.

If you integrate some of these activities into your normal way of living and they eventually become your habits, you will find that your general stress levels decrease. High stress levels are more likely to lead you to seek immediate gratification with alcohol, drugs, or sweet or processed foods. By damping down those stress levels and learning to control anxiety, you will find that your willpower to resist instant gratification is strengthened immeasurably.

Measuring Stress

Recently there have been major advances in our ability to measure the amount of stress that someone is experiencing.

When we breathe in, the stress nerves (activating the sympathetic nervous system) make our heart rate increase; and when we breathe out, the relaxation nerves (activating the parasympathetic nervous system) slow the heart. This means that our heart rates are never even, there is always some variability between beats. If you have a heart rate of 60bpm, that does not mean that your heart beats at exactly 1-second intervals. For example, sometimes the interval between beats could be 0.9 seconds and for other beats 1.1 seconds. When we are tired or particularly stressed, our relaxation and stress nervous systems become fatigued and the variability between heartbeats decreases. If we are fully fit, well rested and not anxious, these nervous systems work well and the variability increases. This is a sign of good health.

Advances in technology mean that there are now many devices that can measure heart rate variability (HRV). The most advanced devices measure HRV when you are in deep sleep and then feed back to you the next day how your body is coping. Many sportspeople use these devices to tell them when they are training too hard. The leading company in this field is called Whoop – their wristband has been worn by many athletes including LeBron James and Rory McIlroy, but it is also a good addition even if you just want to monitor your stress levels.

Hunger

All animals, including humans, have a built-in hunger gauge. Just like the fuel gauge on a car, this internal hunger meter reminds us to fill up when the body senses that our energy levels are low. In humans, the hunger signal comes predominantly from a hormone secreted by the stomach called ghrelin (as we saw in the first chapter, on different hunger hormones). It acts as our reminder to fill up, and the longer we go without food the stronger the hunger signal becomes. We know from the famous Minnesota Starvation Experiment that the signal can become very strong. In this study, a group of young men volunteered to be monitored while consuming a 1,500kcal/day restricted diet, combined with hard physical exercise. Over twenty-four weeks they lost around a quarter of their weight. During the study, their calorie restriction became so extreme that they were unable to concentrate on anything else apart from the prospect of their next meal. Their dreams and fantasies consisted of food, and they stared at food magazines and cookbooks for hours.

The Minnesota study demonstrated the effects of *starvation*, at the extreme end of hunger. However, although we use the word 'starving' in our everyday language, thankfully it is highly unlikely that most of us will ever experience it. However, our hunger signals – and particularly how we read and act on them – are still important when it comes to diet, so let's take a closer look.

Hunger should be seen not as an unpleasant feeling to be avoided, but as a signal that it is soon time to eat – one of the most pleasurable experiences in our day. The hungrier we become, the more enjoyable our meal will be. As hunger increases, so our taste is intensified. The famous phrase 'Hunger is the best sauce' – first written 2,400 years ago – remains relevant today.

Commonly, we mindlessly eat to de-stress even when we are not hungry in the slightest. As we gain more control over our stress levels (perhaps using some of the techniques we've just discussed), so our urge to mindlessly eat should decrease. We can then differentiate between the genuine pleasure of eating natural food in response to hunger versus the false pleasure of eating synthetic food for a dopamine reward.

Here are some ideas for developing a more controlled response to hunger in your daily life . . .

Hunger Scale

It is useful to become aware of your own hunger meter and start to eat in response to it. To make it easier to visualize, let's think again of a fuel gauge on a car. The lowest level is when we are running on empty, the type of hunger we might have after a daylong fast; the highest level is the type of fullness we might feel after a Christmas or Thanksgiving dinner.

The level in the middle is when our hunger is satisfied. One notch down is when we feel slight hunger. You should savour this feeling, and not eat as soon as you feel it. Once the hunger gauge reaches true hunger, it is time to eat and enjoy the pleasure that the food gives you. Some guidance suggests eating to 80 per cent of your satiety (i.e. don't stuff yourself to 100 per cent). You should eat slowly, if possible, and while eating be mindful of your hunger gauge. Once your hunger is satisfied, it is best to stop eating. Fifteen minutes later you should feel fully satisfied as the hormones from your intestines (PYY, GLP-1) signal satiety in your brain. Do not overeat to become uncomfortably full or bloated. You should be able to perform your daily or work tasks after eating. If you need an after-dinner lie-down, it means that you have eaten too much.

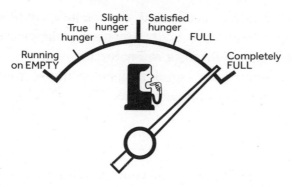

Figure 21: Hunger gauge

Start eating only when truly hungry, and stop eating a meal once your hunger is satisfied.

Time-Restricted Eating

Fasting for as long as is comfortable is good for us, as it decreases stress and inflammation and, if performed regularly, can help us to live for longer. Any prolonged fast will reduce insulin levels and, as we know, insulin is one of the main culprits in blocking our natural weight-control signals (from leptin). When insulin is reduced by fasting, then leptin is no longer blocked and finally our brain can see if we have too much fat stored and it can act to reduce this if it is excessive. This is why *time-restricted eating*, which limits your normal eating period during the day to eight hours or even six hours (named 16:8 or 18:6 eating after the fasting to eating ratio) remains a popular method of weight loss – remember it's not cutting the calories that causes weight loss after regular fasts, it's the effect the fasts have on lowering insulin levels to a more natural level and thereby restoring our normal channels of healthy weight regulation.

Most of us would like to eat as part of a routine of breakfast (if needed), lunch and dinner. If we consume two or three meals per day there is plenty of time between meals to develop true hunger and really enjoy our natural food. In the evening, it is beneficial for your insulin balance not to eat too late or snack after dinner. For instance, you could set yourself a time limit of 9 p.m. to stop eating for the day. This form of time restriction on your eating can be a healthy habit to develop.

During Ramadan, a quarter of the world's population refrain from eating or drinking from sunrise to sunset for a lunar month. The long fasts are not easy, but they teach Muslims the importance of willpower and self-control, make them more mindful of the gifts of God (particularly food when they break their fast), and act as a reminder of the suffering of the poor.

Crave Surfing

Sometimes the urge to do something that is bad for us in the immediate moment overrides the logic to delay gratification. When a craving to perform an addictive and unhealthy habit (like gorging on processed foods) arises, ask yourself how you really feel – question where the craving has come from. By thinking more deeply about the craving and why it has arisen, you can be more mindful in your response – many cravings will pass after a few minutes. A great way to try to stay in control when a craving such as intense hunger begins is a technique called *crave surfing*. Concentrate on your breathing and be mindful of how the craving feels, observing the intensity of the craving as it gets bigger and bigger, like a wave, until it peaks and then crashes. An awareness that cravings get stronger before eventually receding can be an empowering tool.

Ask the Simple Question

A highly effective technique to motivate yourself to perform (or not perform) an action is to ask yourself the simple question 'Am I going to do_____?' For instance, if you are procrastinating about going for a run you can ask yourself simply 'Am I going for a run today?' The question needs to be answered either 'yes' or 'no'. By asking yourself this question, you are clarifying your intrinsic motivation to perform an action. Is this action aligned with your real identity – will it reinforce you? A similar question can be asked in the context of a negative habit or action: 'Am I going to eat junk food tonight?' The answer 'yes' is uncomfortable if the person you are or the person you are becoming is not someone who eats junk food.

Change and Control

We have learned in this chapter that it's much easier to achieve a goal of weight loss or improved health if the habit changes needed for this align with our true identity. Once we under stand how our food environment affects our health, our identity is open to change and we can adapt who we really are and how we react to situations. This change creates a natural aversion to unhealthy processed foods and a desire for more natural healthy foods. Minimal willpower is needed to change.

By understanding how we can be triggered into bad habits and how to overwrite these habits with ones that are better for us, we can make real progress in improving the routines in our lives. Changing our surroundings, or the people we interact with, can increase the friction to perform a bad habit and make better habits easier to perform. Repetition of a good habit, even if the action or activity itself is only for a short period of time, is crucial in order to embed it into our brains.

Stress can cause us to seek out a reward to make us feel transiently better, but often these 'rewards' are bad for us. Eating processed foods for reward rather than for hunger changes them into a type of damaging drug, making us feel transiently better but harming our health. By controlling our stress, we can more easily control our desire for instant gratification.

Back on the Road to Glasgow – a Year Later

The long journey to Glasgow for the start of my daughter's second year at university was a wholly different and much more satisfying experience from a culinary point of view. This time we had planned not just the start time, but the location of our stops and the types of food that we would eat along the way. It took preparation, but we both felt a lot better physically at the end of our journey.

This time, the sun was shining for most of the way, and instead of being corralled into a grimy service station for a toxic breakfast we found ourselves sitting on a picnic bench in a national park. We had prepared a traditional Japanese breakfast of crispy teriyaki salmon, sticky rice in small bowls, home-made pickled cucumber, carrot and ginger, and miso soup. As we savoured our food and poured green tea from our flask, the thought of eating fast food was never further from our minds. The cravings had passed.

CHAPTER 10

Cookery School

'Let food be thy medicine and medicine be thy food.'

Hippocrates

McDonald's, Southampton High Street, Saturday Afternoon, June 1988

The eight burgers sizzled instantly as I carefully placed them on the red-hot grill and pressed the 30-second timer button.

'CHEESE ON FIVE!!' shouted my supervisor, his voice getting more high-pitched as the restaurant filled and the queue lengthened. I readied the five artificial cheese squares. As the buzzer sounded, I flipped the burgers over and placed the cheese over five of them, pressing my timer again. My assistant had the toasted, sugar-infused buns ready. BEEP-BEEP-BEEP ... I quickly transferred the browned and aromatic burgers onto the buns while she carefully added the thin layer of ketchup, the gherkin and the sesame bun top, before closing it in the brightly coloured cardboard box.

Twenty minutes of burger-flipping later and I was on my only break in the ten-hour shift. Employees were allowed to eat as much food as they could during their break, just so long as it had passed its strict sell-by time, meaning it would have been disposed of otherwise. I grabbed two burgers, an order of fries,

195

three apple pies and a large chocolate shake. Downstairs, my fellow workers and I sat in the small dingy basement, devouring our trays of fast food like a silent pack of wild animals, intent on eating as much as we could in as little time as possible.

But by day ten in the job, the thought of another burger made me feel sick, my body felt weak and bloated, and an eruption of acne covered my face . . . Needless to say, I didn't last much longer in my first role as a cook.

My first real interest in cooking came in my third year of medical school. I was fortunate enough to be part of a large house-share with a group of Indian friends. Unlike me, who had never been taught to cook, my friends took great pleasure in cooking fantastically tasty fresh Indian food on a regular basis. Where I had only seen a 'curry' cooked with curry powder, they used fresh spices. Finely chopped garlic, ginger, onion and chilli were sautéed, and garam masala and turmeric powder were added. Cumin seeds, cardamom pods, nutmeg, star anise and curry leaves all followed, giving off a swirl of wonderful aromas. The concoctions might include chicken or lamb, served alongside vegetable dishes using colourful sweet peppers, ripe tomatoes, potatoes and gorgeous okra. Perfectly cooked rice, a yogurt and cucumber raita, a pot of dhal, and a simple onion-based salad would cover our table as we savoured the delicious food while we joked around, telling our stories from the day.

Since learning to cook from my Indian friends, I have continued, wherever possible, to learn new dishes and experience other cuisines throughout the world, including the Caribbean, Brazil, Costa Rica, India, Thailand and many parts of Africa and the Arab world. I have picked up new ideas and cooking techniques in recent years using fresh-food meal-kit deliveries, and my daughters and I now know our way around many fantastic global dishes. The purpose of this book is in part to encourage people to embrace real food and to experience the globe's wide variety of cuisines, so in the coming chapters I have set out some key techniques, ingredients and advice for those who have never cooked from scratch before, or who want to increase the number of natural foods they eat and cook with on a regular basis. We are blessed in our current age to be able to access many different types of ingredients. Whether we prefer South Asian or Middle Eastern cuisines, Brazilian or Japanese, we can now choose to prepare our own favourite dishes that originate from anywhere in the world.

Preparing delicious meals from fresh ingredients is not only better in terms of taste, it also comes with powerful health benefits. The international recipes and suggestions in chapter 12, Global Kitchen, are specially chosen to help reset your weight. The nutrition they provide is designed to have a profoundly healthy effect on your body, leading to efficient insulin signalling, decreased inflammation, and the seamless shedding of excess fat. Once cooking foods like these becomes a habit, it will feel like you have a new, highly efficient body.

Before we enter the kitchen, I have a disclaimer to make. I am not a cook or a chef, and I have never had any formal culinary training. The advice that follows therefore comes from an enthusiastic amateur's perspective only. Please feel free to skip sections if you feel confident in these areas already, though I hope that even keen chefs will find something here worthy of their further thought.

What to Avoid

It's important to remember the recommendations of what to eat and what to avoid. We have learned that *sugar* and *refined carbohydrates* stimulate the weight-gain trigger by blocking the leptin signal that the brain uses to gauge the amount of fat you are carrying. In addition, *fructose*, the sugar that comes from fruit, can cause a separate weight-gain trigger similar to an animal's hibernation state when ingested in large amounts. Fresh fruits are fine in moderation, but fruit juices of any kind can stimulate this weight-gain trigger, and we know that processed foods are infused with this addictive ultra-sweet additive. Finally, *vegetable oils* of any kind are not natural human foods. They massively disrupt our internal metabolic balance, which is why my ten-day vegetable-oil-infused McDonald's binge when I worked there made me feel so unwell. The omega-6 fatty acids in these oils coat every cell in our bodies, diluting the health-giving omega-3 fatty acids found in fresh foods, and causing inflammation and misfiring our insulin, meaning more insulin is needed. For our bodies, it's like taking a massive extra sugar and inflammatory hit, but without the sugar or the cellular injury.

A note of caution regarding foods to avoid that contain large amounts of omega-6. Unfortunately, it is not just fried fast foods and processed foods that contain too much of this fat. Any animal that has consumed unnaturally high levels of omega-6 will itself contain large amounts. Just like humans, animals that have been (farm) fed on grains and seeds grow faster and are fatter than if fed their natural diet. Almost all chickens, even if allowed to live in a field, will have been grown on grains and will have unnaturally high amounts of omega-6. A truly wild chicken will roam around eating worms and insects, but these chickens are slim and wiry and will not interest any supermarket. The same can be said of hens' eggs. The yolk of the egg has high omega-6 levels, and therefore if you want to normalize the omega fats in your own body opt for egg whites,* which are a great protein source. Other farm-fed animal meats that should be avoided are pork and grain-fed beef. The good news is that wild fish, grass-fed beef and lamb have a healthy omega-fat profile and can be savoured and enjoyed. In summary, avoid:

- *All processed foods* whose *main* ingredients are the poisonous trinity of sugar, artificial fructose sweeteners and vegetable oils.
- *Foods whose main ingredient is sugar*, though the odd teaspoon in cooking is acceptable.
- *Refined carbohydrates* such as wheat flour. Again they're OK in cooking as an additive to sauces and as a crispy coating.
- *Vegetable oils*, including sunflower oil, rapeseed oil, corn oil, cottonseed oil, safflower oil, 'vegetable' oil, canola oil (ignore the 'high in omega-3 claim' – it disappears within thirty seconds of heating), margarine, 'easy spread' fake butter and shortening. These oils should not be allowed anywhere near your kitchen. They also infuse all fast food (because they can cook at high heat), processed foods (because they don't oxidize easily and so have a long shelf life), and farm-fattened meat including chicken, pork and grain-fed beef. It will take at least six months for your body to be cleansed of the omega-6 from these oils already clinging to your cells. Once cleansed, you will feel much better.

---

* Many people worried about the high cholesterol level of egg yolks have been doing this for years. We now know that it's not the cholesterol in the egg yolk that causes inflammation, cardiac risk and obesity; it's the omega-6 fats contained in them.

Different people seek different outcomes for their health, and you will need to adapt your diet to your needs. If you would like to lose weight (and improve type 2 diabetes, high blood pressure, high cholesterol, and heart disease) then, in addition to avoiding processed foods, sugar and vegetable oils, you will also need to be cautious of consuming too many carbs in the form of white rice, potatoes and home-baked breads. My first book, *Why We Eat (Too Much)*, charts the amount of carbohydrate in most common foods, but if you are aware of your portion size (smaller plates) and your hunger (not eating to beyond fullness), limiting carbohydrate intake should prove simple.

Remember that if you do a lot of physical activity, you will need more food, and as long as it's prepared from fresh ingredients this is OK. If your aim is primarily to improve your long-term health and avoid or improve modern inflammatory diseases such as asthma, eczema, psoriasis, inflammatory bowel disease, rheumatoid arthritis and fibromyalgia, you don't need to watch out particularly for your natural carbohydrate intake – cutting sugar and avoiding processed food and vegetable oils will suffice.

What to Eat

This leaves the foods to eat. Essentially, you can choose any foods that are not in the above categories. Remember that fresh vegetables, particularly leafy green and brightly coloured ones, infuse your body with phytochemicals, those anti-inflammatory and life-extending antioxidant messages from our plant friends. They provide carbohydrates in amounts that are natural to our bodies. Taking in most of your carbohydrates via these types of vegetables is highly recommended. If you do this, your body will reactivate your normal weight-control mechanisms and excess fat will be sensed and shed.

Fish that are not farmed will be overflowing with omega-3, priming your body to reduce inflammation and improving weight control by reducing insulin requirements.

Red meat is *not* bad for you. It is full of health-giving natural saturated fats. These fats do not spike insulin levels and do not cause obesity. Grass-fed meat (beef and lamb) is better as it will have higher omega-3 levels. Chicken and pork, although deemed by many nutritionists to be good for you (because of the misplaced belief that low saturated fat is good) are usually farm-fed on grains that are high in the pro-inflammatory omega-6, meaning they also contain high amounts of this toxic fat.

Pulses and beans are a fantastic source of healthy high-protein calories and can be used in place of typical staple carbs (rice, pasta, potato). Another often overlooked alternative to traditional carbohydrates is grains like buckwheat or quinoa. They are easy to prepare, tasty, have lower effects on insulin, and feature higher protein and nutrient contents compared to traditional carbs. If you switch to these foods instead of rice, your body will respond favourably.

Eggplant, also known as aubergine, is easy to cook and again can replace traditional carbs in a meal. The best fruits to consume are berries, which are full of phytochemicals and low in fructose sugar.

If you consume dairy products, natural yogurts and cottage cheeses are high in protein, calcium and B vitamins. These are great foods to start your day with.

A Note on Saturated Fat

The research linking cholesterol to heart disease in the 1960s and '70s has subsequently been proven to be wrong. As long as you don't have a rare condition called familial hypercholesterolaemia, where blood cholesterol levels are extremely high, you do not need to avoid foods containing cholesterol or natural saturated fat. There is no link between the amount of these fats consumed and the risk of cardiac disease.

In fact, when the US and UK populations were told to stop eating so many of these fats and switch to grains and more sugary foods, they started to develop obesity and diabetes. So, the message is it's OK to eat fatty steaks and red meat, butter, yogurt and some natural cheese. The only saturated fat to avoid is palm oil, which does cause problems with heart disease. Palm oil has found its way into a lot of processed food (as it is cheap and gives good mouthfeel), and it's best to avoid cooking or ingesting this oil wherever possible.

In summary, imagine the natural foods that are available at your butcher's, fishmonger's and greengrocer's. These foods are very good for your health. If your aim is health rather than weight loss, then bread – if home-baked from wholegrain flour – can be eaten in moderation. Remember that supermarket bread is ultra-processed and should therefore be avoided if possible.

Preparing Your Kitchen

Remember that your environment plays a big part in whether you will perform an action or not, and whether you will form good or bad habits. A badly organized and equipped kitchen, and a poorly stocked pantry, will make it much less likely that you will enjoy cooking great food. The first step is to clear your kitchen surfaces of all non-kitchen clutter and of any equipment that you rarely use. Declutter the novelty cutting devices and any large bulky appliances that you don't use regularly, such as the coffee machine or juicer. Store them away and get them out when needed. This should create more counter-top space. Throw away, or recycle, chipped mugs and plates and fading plastic containers. Check the food items in the fridge and pantry, and throw away anything that has passed its use-by date or has been open too long. Everything should be as fresh as possible. Get rid of your vegetable oils (they are not food) and any jars of sauces, mixes or dips that contains lots of these oils.

You will need the following essential kitchen equipment:

- Chopping board – the size should suit the size of the worktop space you have. I prefer a large, sturdy, heavy wooden one (like a butcher's block), but many people use plastic. To stop a kitchen board slipping when you are using it, place a damp kitchen towel underneath it.
- Chef's knife – you will have seen the famous TV chefs wielding these big, heavy, sharp-pointed knives. They have a sloping curved blade, which facilitates the signature rocking motion when cutting and chopping.

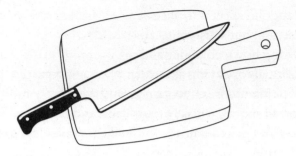

Figure 22: Chef's knife

- Knife sharpener – there is nothing more pleasurable than cutting with a razor-sharp knife, and nothing more frustrating than a blunt one. A handheld pull-through sharpener or a steel honing rod are the simplest options. Electric sharpeners are convenient and really work, but take up space. My personal favourite is the old-fashioned whetstone sharpener.
- Small paring knife – like a chef's knife but smaller. Great for chopping onions, garlic and ginger, or peeling fresh fruits.
- Serrated knife – to cut food that has a thick surface such as (home-made) crusty bread, and tomatoes.
- Meat cleaver or Chinese cleaver – to chop meat into smaller portions and for the easy chopping of large, tough vegetables.
- Swivel peeler – for potatoes.
- Box grater – for carrots, vegetables and cheese.
- Fine grater – for parmesan, nutmeg, citrus zest and ginger.

- Mandolin slicer – to slice vegetables very finely. Not essential but satisfying to use.
- Mixing bowl, colander and salad spinner – the latter is essential for drying and storing washed lettuce.
- Cooking utensils – wooden spoon, tongs, spatula, slotted spoon, whisk, masher, mortar and pestle.
- Pots and pans – a non-stick frying pan (skillet), and selection of different-sized saucepans.
- Cast-iron griddle pan – this is perhaps not essential, but griddling makes cooking fun.
- Roasting and baking trays.
- Stick blender – plus a tall mixing jug or beaker.
- Kitchen scales – the electronic versions are easiest.

On the Dinner Table

In the 1960s, our plates measured around 8.5 inches (22cm) and could hold 800kcal of food. Over the past few decades, plate sizes have increased more and more. Today's plates measure 12 inches (30cm) and can hold around 1,900kcal. Rather than using these modern large plates, I would recommend going retro and using the plate sizes of the 1960s. By using the smaller plate you are more likely to eat slower, enjoy your food and stop when you are no longer hungry. A larger plate encourages overeating.

A chopping board can double up as a serving board. Food can be placed on the table so your family and friends can serve themselves. If you are trying to cut down on carbs, leave the bowls containing them furthest from reach or in the kitchen once you have served, so that it takes more effort to get seconds.

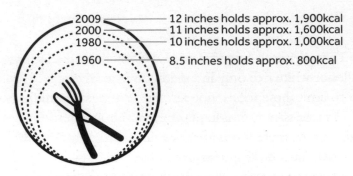

2009 ——————— 12 inches holds approx. 1,900kcal
2000 ————— 11 inches holds approx. 1,600kcal
1980 ————— 10 inches holds approx. 1,000kcal
1960 ————— 8.5 inches holds approx. 800kcal

Figure 23: Dinner plates 1960s to now

Storage

A well-organized kitchen needs lots of different-sized Tupperware with a secure locking mechanism to avoid leaks and spills. It is best to take your lunch with you if you are going to be out of the house, to avoid unhealthy high-street options, so these containers are essential.

Freezer bags and plastic boxes with lids can be used to freeze excess food that you have cooked, to eat another day. Small pots and jars come in useful for storing your spice mixes and home-made pickles.

Preparing Your Pantry

Remember that you are now taking control of your food. This means that you are no longer reliant on short-term convenience meals, fast foods or deliveries. Your kitchen pantry should be fully stocked with non-perishable items that can easily be combined with fresh food to help make a wide array of dishes. Having a well-stocked pantry will make cooking much easier, and make it more likely that cooking becomes your normal habit.

Grains and Pulses

If you are trying to lose weight, I would advise eating pasta, noodles or white rice only in moderation – or if you find it difficult to limit these foods, not storing them in your kitchen at all. If weight is not an issue and your aim is just to become healthier, then these foods are acceptable. Either way, healthier alternatives include bulgur wheat, couscous, quinoa, wild rice, brown rice and soba noodles (made from buckwheat).

Pulses are high in protein and fibre. They can be stored dried or tinned. Depending on your taste, pulses to have stored might include: red split lentils, kidney beans, black beans, split peas, chickpeas, cannellini beans and mixed beans.

Tinned and Dried Foods

Chopped tomatoes and coconut milk are versatile additions to many dishes, and water chestnuts are a great ingredient in stir-fries.

Canned fish such as tuna, salmon, sardines or mackerel (in tomato, and not oil) are convenient snacks that are full of nutrients, particularly omega-3. Canned anchovies can be used to add a salty and protein taste to dishes.

Canned fruit should be in water and not syrup. Canned fruits lose some phytochemical goodness but remain a reasonable (and longer lasting) alternative to fresh fruits. Pineapple chunks are a good addition to add a tangy sweetness to some dishes.

Vinegars and Oils

Red and white wine vinegar, rice wine vinegar, mirin and balsamic vinegar can be added to a dish towards the end of cooking.

The acidic taste stimulates the 'sour' receptors in the tongue to give a more complete taste experience. Plain white vinegar can be used to make your own pickles. Sherry can be used to add a sweet flavour to dishes.

Instead of vegetable oils, stock your pantry with extra-virgin olive oil, butter, coconut butter and clarified butter (ghee). Olive oil (in bottles) should not be left out as it will be degraded by sunlight, so store it away to prolong its freshness.

Sauces and Condiments

These might include Dijon and English mustard (these can also be used as emulsifying agents in home-made sauces), soy sauce, teriyaki sauce, Worcestershire sauce, pepper sauce and sriracha sauce.

Pickles

Capers add a tangy, lemon / olive burst of flavour to dishes, particularly fish and pasta sauces. Dill pickles and olives are great to have on hand for an antipasto platter. Don't forget that fresh pickles can be easily made at home – pickled red onions, small cucumbers (dill pickles), carrots, radishes, and red and white cabbage are great sources of vitamins (A, B and C) and healing phytochemicals.

Frozen Food Essentials

A well-stocked freezer is an important part of your kitchen. Frozen fruits and vegetables are not only cheaper than fresh, but they are also frozen as soon as they are picked – meaning they are fresh when cooked and retain all their phytochemical goodness. Prawns don't need to be defrosted before cooking, and sea fish such as cod, haddock and sea bass – which are frozen minutes after they are caught, meaning they are ultra-fresh – can easily be baked from frozen.

Preparing Your Spice Rack

Unlike the E-number spice rack described in chapter 2 – full of toxic chemicals with artificial flavours, emulsifiers and colourings – your natural spice rack is a nutritional power-house containing minerals, vitamins and those important anti-inflammatory phytochemicals. This is because your cooking spices originate from our plant friends.

A fully stocked spice section in your kitchen is essential in order to impart layers of wonderful aromas, flavours and taste to your meals.

Spices come in the form of whole seeds (cumin seeds, carda-mom pods, peppercorns) or ground spices. Whole seeds can retain their flavour for longer, up to 2–3 years, however once the seeds are cracked and ground into powder, their oils – which contain distinctive flavours and aromas – are exposed to the air and oxygen starts to degrade their flavour. Ground spices have a shorter shelf life of around six months. After this time they should be replaced with freshly ground aromatic spices. They should be stored away from sunlight.

As you are cooking and adding different spices to your dish, make a habit of regularly tasting the changing flavours, as this helps you gain familiarity and confidence.

Some recommended spices to have at hand include:

- *Pepper*, either whole or ground. Whole peppercorns retain a stronger spicy taste than ground black pepper. White pepper is hotter but has a less complex flavour than black pepper. White pepper is commonly used in place of black pepper in soups and chowders to avoid unsightly black specks.
- *Cumin* is a beautifully earthy and sweet aromatic spice used in cuisines from India, North Africa, the Middle East, Southern Europe and Mexico. Cumin seeds are harvested from a plant in the parsley family. Cumin can be added – in the form of either seeds or ground spice – at the start of cooking to flavour an oil, to food during cooking, as an ingredient in a marinade, or to yogurt in a raita, or simply sprinkled over roasted vegetables or salads.
- *Cardamom*, whole or ground. This spice has a distinctive sweet and peppery flavour, and originates from a plant in the ginger family found in India and Sri Lanka. It is used in aromatic curries and sometimes baking.
- *Fresh or dried chillies*, when added to food, increase its mouthfeel. The typical burning sensation in the mouth that chillies give adds to the flavour experience. Chillies have been linked to increased metabolism and weight loss.
- *Chilli powder* is a blend of spices that includes powder from dried chillies, combined with savoury spices such as cumin, garlic powder, onion powder and paprika.
- *Cayenne pepper* is made solely from hot cayenne peppers that have been dried and ground. It is extremely hot compared to chilli powder.

- *Paprika* originates from the capsicum (sweet) peppers of Mexico. A mix of milder and stronger peppers are commonly used, meaning the heat is variable. It gives a sweet, earthy, peppery taste to foods, and lights them up with a deep red colour. It is commonly used in casseroles and to make barbecue sauces, and can be sprinkled on soup and egg dishes.
- *Chilli flakes* are made from dried red peppers, usually the cayenne variety of hot pepper. Like cayenne powder, they have a much stronger chilli heat than chilli powder.
- *Coriander* (seeds or ground spice) has a sweet, slightly lemony flavour. It complements cumin wonderfully, and these two spices are often mixed to form the base of a spice blend.
- *Turmeric* has been used in both cooking and medicine for centuries. Its main constituent, curcumin, is a powerful heath-giving anti-inflammatory phytochemical. It is extracted from the roots of a plant in the ginger family (fresh turmeric looks similar to fresh ginger). It imparts a deep yellow colour to food. Make sure that the powder is fresh to maximize its health benefits.
- *Fenugreek* seeds or leaves are an essential addition to many curry dishes, providing excellent antioxidant health benefits and imparting a bitter maple-syrup-like flavour and aroma if added towards the end of cooking.
- *Star anise* is the dried fruit and seed of evergreen trees native to regions of Vietnam and China. Although not related to aniseed, it has a similar taste. Its sweet liquorice flavour is mainly used for soups, broths, curries and tea.

- *Cinnamon* (whole stick or ground) originates from the bark of cinnamon trees in Sri Lanka. It imparts a sweet and smoky taste to foods, and adds deep flavour to savoury dishes from around the world. It is also commonly used in baking.
- *Nutmeg* lends an earthy, nutty and sweet flavour to both sweet and savoury dishes.
- *Cloves* are often used alongside cinnamon and nutmeg in sweet dishes. They have a pungent, sweet taste, similar to cinnamon, and are responsible for 'the smell of Christmas' when added to mulled wines or roast ham. Cloves are present in Chinese five-spice and Indian garam masala blends.

Remember, fresh spices make food taste great. They are an essential part of eating and living well. Get to know their flavours and how they can be combined, and fresh, tasty foods will become a welcome part of your cooking routine, ultimately improving your weight and your health.

Spice Blends

Finding the correct spice combinations takes time and cooking practice. The more you cook, the more experienced you will become. To make things easier, there are many spice blends available. These are specially prepared to include specific ground spices, in the correct proportions for different cuisines. Examples are Italian herb seasoning, garam masala and chaat masala (for Indian flavours), five-spice (Chinese), za'atar (Middle Eastern), ras el hanout (Morocco), berbere (Ethiopian) and shichimi togarashi (Japanese seven-spice).

You can try making your own spice blends using combinations

of whole spices. Use either a pestle and mortar or a spice grinder to release the natural flavours and aromatic oils of the spice seeds as they are ground down. These totally unique mixes can be stored for weeks, but the sooner you use them the fresher the flavour will be.

Dried Herbs

Dried oregano is used in Italian and Mexican cuisines, and is great with tomato- and cheese-based dishes. Bay leaves, thyme and basil add a savoury sweetness and aroma to stews and soups, and dried rosemary gives its distinctive flavour to roasted meats and to slow-cooked casseroles. Dried mint can be used to add its subtle sweetness and freshness to chicken and lamb marinades or pea soup, and can be sprinkled on finely diced Middle Eastern salads.

Fresh Herbs

Rather than buying fresh herbs from the supermarket that will only last a few days, it's better (if you have the time) to have a variety of home-grown herb plants available in your kitchen. These can be grown from seed or bought as small plants. Herbs that grow well indoors and are useful in many different dishes include basil, mint, oregano, chives, rosemary and parsley.

As we know from chapter 5, plants only need some water and a good amount of light to convert that CO_2 in the air into growth. They need to be located next to a window that gets many hours of sunlight (preferably south-facing if you are in the northern hemisphere). Don't overwater indoor herbs. Once they reach around 15cm (6 inches) tall, encourage more growth by occasionally trimming some leaves, even if you don't need them for cooking. In this way, they will thrive.

Salt

Salt should be recognized as the most important 'spice' in cooking. When added to food, it does not just make that food taste saltier, it unlocks other flavours and aromas and the spices that have been added. As Samin Nosrat says in her book *Salt Fat Acid Heat*, without salt, food would be 'adrift in a sea of blandness'.

It really does have a greater impact on flavour than any other ingredient. The term 'season to taste' refers mainly to salt. As you are cooking, keep tasting your food, and add a little salt to a spoonful of it and see if flavours are amplified and improved. Your food should taste not overtly salty but certainly not bland; you should add enough to make the flavours of the food burst out.

Salt also blunts bitter tastes in food and can be a better alternative to sugar when trying to sweeten bitter flavours. Unless you suffer from high blood pressure or kidney problems, the amount of salt that you use in your cooking should not be an issue.

Not all salt is the same or has the same taste, however. Table salt, common in most kitchens, has iodine added to it, which imparts a metallic taste. In addition, table salt usually contains an artificial anti-caking agent to stop it clumping together and to keep it pouring out smoothly. Sea salt, formed after the evaporation of sea water and containing natural sea minerals, is a better option. Himalayan salt is an alternative to sea salt. It is a pink-coloured rock salt containing traces of magnesium, potassium and calcium, extracted from mines near the Himalayan mountains.

A Note on Salt

Salt is a crucial ingredient for home cooks. It brings out fantastic flavours, particularly in meat and fish dishes. Most chefs want to use salt liberally, but is it safe for our health? For many years there has been a 'war on salt'. Most people think that they should be careful with their intake, and have an understanding that too much salt causes high blood pressure. Government guidelines recommend that we cut our salt intake from the current level of 3.4g to 2.3g per day – the equivalent of a teaspoon of salt. But recent reports suggest salt may not be as dangerous as previously thought.

The whole edifice of research linking salt to high blood pressure is based on experiments from the 1970s. Scientist Lewis Dahl at the Brookhaven National Laboratory in New York fed rats large amounts of salt and observed that their blood pressure rose when he did this, proving a link between the two. However, the amount of salt he had to administer to the rats to get positive results for his trial would be the equivalent of feeding a human 500g of salt per day. That's over 80 tsp of salt!

Recent analysis of several large trials looking at the effect of limiting salt intake on health in 6,250 people found that there was zero evidence that cutting salt reduces the risk of hypertension, heart disease or stroke. A further study found that people who excreted *less* salt from their kidneys (because they had consumed less) had a *higher* risk of dying from a heart attack. More recently, the focus has shifted towards processed foods as causal in high blood pressure and heart disease. But it doesn't seem to be the salt in these foods that cause the health risks; it is more likely to be the very industrial quantities of added sugar, particularly sweet fructose sugar, that they contain.

Meal Planning

Planning ahead will make your cooking experience easier and more enjoyable. Have a list of your favourite recipes to hand when you plan your weekly meals. This list should regularly be added to as you learn how to cook more and more dishes.

Take a look in your (and your family's) diary to identify the days that you won't need to cook. Choose your recipes for the week and write out the ingredients that you will need for these (checking what you currently have). Your grocery shopping should ideally be when you have time and are not rushed or stressed. You might want to get even fresher groceries from a farmers' market, or you could check for online fresh-food delivery services. There are now many companies, such as Oddbox and Riverford (in the UK), who will deliver fresh picked fruits and vegetables to your door. There are other online companies that can deliver high-quality frozen meats and fish.

You may also consider using a meal-kit delivery company such as Gousto, Hello Fresh or Mindful Chef for some of your evening meals. They deliver just the right amount of ingredients and spices/herbs in one box, with easy-to-follow cooking instructions, and make learning new cooking techniques and dishes fun.

Tips before Starting

Read the recipe of the meal that you are going to cook, and gather all the ingredients and spices that you will need. Make sure your cooking utensils are ready. Don't be shy to swap out ingredients if a particular one is not available. If you are not very experienced in the kitchen, remember that the more you cook the better you will get at it, just like with any skill. Don't become disheartened if your meal doesn't look or taste the way you had hoped. Learn as you cook – trial and error is OK.

Cooking Skills

To become confident at cooking it is useful to learn some new skills. These can be learned from a cookery class, or these days more easily from the numerous helpful YouTube videos on the subject. There are several skills that are incredibly helpful to learn . . .

Knife skills are essential to becoming a better cook, as they form the basis of all cooking and are something you will use every day. Mostly you will be using your large chef's knife. Grip the knife close to the blade. Cutting vegetables should not be as a chopping action but a rocking motion, like a wave. Cutting skills that are useful to master include *dicing, mincing, chiffonade* (cutting leafy greens into ribbons) and *julienning* (cutting foods into matchstick-shaped pieces).

Sautéing is the process of cooking food quickly in a small amount of fat over a high heat. Make sure the pan is very hot before you add your cooking oil by splashing a few drops of water on it to check the heat. The water should fizz and evaporate quickly. The oil should have a high smoke point, so clarified butter (ghee) is preferable to olive oil for this method of cooking (or avocado oil if you are vegan). As the food cooks, it should be turned in the pan regularly with a sautéing or jumping motion (*sauté* in French means 'jumped'). The motion is a little like flipping a pancake.

Roasting is a method of cooking food in the oven using dry heat and very hot air. With this method, food is cooked evenly in all directions. There are three important stages in roasting food: *searing*, where the food is browned on the outside, creating wonderful flavours; *cooking*, where the food is left at the correct heat and for the correct duration to cook all the way through; and *resting* (for roasted meats), to give time for the juices to redistribute within the meat and make carving easier.

Caramelization and Browning

Every good chef knows the importance of two types of chemical reaction that can occur when cooking foods at high temperatures: the *Maillard reaction* and *caramelization*.

When roasting, sautéing or barbecuing any food that contains sugars and proteins, the Maillard reaction will occur at a temperature of around 150 °C (300 °F). The amino acids and sugars on the outer layer of the food undergo a chemical reaction, causing a brown pigmentation to form and the release of protein flavour compounds – giving a great taste and smell to the food (think of the smell of a roast joint or a barbecue). Searing meat before roasting it adds extra flavour using this reaction. Other foods that brown in this way are fried steak, baked bread crust, coffee beans, and the tasty brown underside of fried eggs.

Caramelization occurs when foods containing sugar are cooked over a low heat. The sugar in the food oxidizes and browns, changing its taste to a sweet, nutty caramel flavour. Examples of this are the roof of a crème brûlée after the sugar has been gently heated with a blowtorch, and caramelized onions, which are slowly fried in a pan until sweet and brown.

Emulsification is the process of combining water- and oil-based liquids, usually in a freshly made sauce. This process is used extensively in processed foods using artificial ingredients, but it is also an essential cooking skill to use in your own kitchen. Oil and water do not mix; even if they are shaken or whisked together it will not be long before they separate. Natural emulsifying ingredients work as the middle man, holding on to both water-based and oil-based liquids and therefore forming an emulsion – a mixture of two liquids that would not normally mix together. A good example of this is oil and vinegar. To mix these together to form a vinaigrette for your salad that will not separate, an emulsifier is needed. In your kitchen the most useful emulsifiers are mustard (particularly Dijon), egg yolks and honey. Add any of these and an emulsion will be formed.

Brining is essential to bring out beautiful flavours, and retain moisture, when cooking meat or fish. When salt infuses into meat (or fish), it causes the protein strands in the muscle to unravel and tangle with other unwound proteins, and this protein 'weave' attracts and retains water. When the meat is cooked, it maintains its moisture – meaning that the meat or fish is much juicier and less likely to be overdone. In addition to keeping the meat more succulent, the salt itself will amplify the flavours and aromas of the food.

Salt should be added quite liberally, so don't use the salt shaker as this will not give enough salt. Pour out a handful of salt and sprinkle over the meat so that most of it is well covered. It will take time for the salt to infuse into the meat. The larger or thicker the meat, the longer is needed for salt to infuse deeply into it. A medium-sized steak can be salted hours before cooking. For whole chickens and joints of meat, brining should start preferably the day before cooking. If you want to brine a large Christmas or Thanksgiving turkey, then you could consider using a sealed brining bag. The water that is added to the bag should have the same taste as seawater – very salty.

Fish absorbs salt much faster than meat. Salting can be done around fifteen minutes before cooking. Use just the right amount of salt and you will really notice how succulent and tasty the fish is.

Taste Combinations and Seasoning

While cooking and tasting your food, remember that our palate likes lots of different flavours together. Salt is the number-one spice and needs to be added in just the right amount to bring out the full flavour of the dish. But remember to add something sweet (ripe tomatoes, pineapple, etc.) and something bitter (lemon, vinegar) to dishes too, as when you do this you will taste the full orchestra of flavours.

Also be aware of mouthfeel – remember we like the contrast of soft and chewy and crunchy foods, as well as oily sauces or emulsions that coat all parts of our mouths.

Finally, be aware of the look of your meal. We humans like colour contrast, and the more brightly coloured foods appear on our plate, the more we will savour our meal.

CHAPTER II

Last Orders

Why Food Matters

Close your eyes and imagine this. You are sitting at a white table in a brightly lit white room. In front of you is a large white plate. Imagine that on this plate is your favourite processed food – perhaps a portion of fried chicken, fries or a burger. Or perhaps it's cake, chocolate or brightly coloured chewy sweets. The plate is overflowing. You are tasked with eating all this food and finishing off the plate. You are not hungry, but even before you start eating you feel good as you notice the bright colours enticing you to devour the food. Imagine yourself chewing this food, mouthful by mouthful, your teeth breaking it up, releasing the artificial emulsifiers to pleasantly coat your tongue with oil, freeing the chemical fla vourings to dance around your mouth until they latch on to the correct taste receptors on your tongue, tricking your brain into liking the food. As the food travels into your digestive system, imagine that you have a sophisticated scanner that allows you to see all the chemical reactions taking place. As the food finds its way into your blood, you can see the sugars and oils blocking your normal appetite regulation as you keep eating. You notice the chemicals from the colourings and fla vourings at war with your immune system throughout your body. Your brain is oblivious to the damage that is being done, still flickering in excitement like a broken lamp. The image pans back out to you taking the last mouthful, feeling queasy and bloated as the food becomes you and you become the food.

In this book, we have learned that processed foods – and any foods containing too much sugar, refined carbohydrates, fructose and vegetable oils – have a terrible effect on our health. They disrupt our normal weight regulation systems and can cause weight gain. When we eat too many of these foods, our weight set-point can increase to an unhealthy level and we end up storing far too many calories as fat. Our brain can't sense the excess fat because the leptin signal that is supposed to inform it of our energy storage status is blocked. Our brain will fight against attempts to lose weight via calorie-counting diets or exercise. Remember, our brain can manipulate our metabolic energy to plummet (by around 600kcal), and it can send us powerful and irresistible appetite signals – suddenly an hour in the gym or a 1,200kcal diet is written off. It's not the calories in the food that trigger weight gain; it's what the food does to our bodies. It's how the brain reads those food signals and shifts our weight anchor to a heavier place. This is why, when we try to lose weight by calorie restriction, it doesn't work long-term. You might think you have won the dietary battle over a few weeks, but your body will win the weight-regain war eventually.

The way to lose weight and keep it off is to be smart, to understand the effects these foods have on your weight regulation system, and to avoid these foods by creating better habits. This means cutting out most processed foods and being aware of and reducing the carbohydrate content of foods by reducing portion size, only eating until satisfied (and not full), and not snacking between meals or in the evening before bed.

It's not just our weight but also our health that is at stake. Ultra-processed foods contain a multitude of artificial chemical additives (preservatives, colourings and flavourings) that have been shown to increase the risk of severe allergies and chronic inflammatory and degenerative conditions such as asthma, painful arthritis, inflammatory bowel conditions and Alzheimer's.

By eating too much processed food, we deprive ourselves of the health-giving anti-inflammatory and antioxidant (anti-ageing) effects that natural foods contain. By reducing our intake of these natural plant medicines, we increase our risk of inflammatory diseases even more.

But cutting out processed foods and sugars is easier said than done. Processed foods are scientifically designed to be wonderful-looking and have appealing flavours. They make us feel great by lighting up our reward pathways. They are specifically designed and marketed so that we can easily become hooked on them. This is what the food companies want – it drives sales and profits. It's easy for bad eating habits to become ingrained in our vulnerable brains, and it's difficult to change these habits.

So how do we change? We should be reassured that we are already changing. Day by day, minute by minute, each one of us is constantly changing our identity. Every time we learn or experience something new, this changes our outlook on the world and the way we react to it. By learning and understanding how damaging processed foods can be and how medicinal fresh foods are for us, we will change. We are less likely to want to consume these foods, but we understand the urges and drives that remind us how good these foods make us feel.

It is likely that, having read this book, your perception of the food environment surrounding you has changed. You are now aware of the mechanism of weight gain and weight loss, as your weight anchor shifts up and down in response to your food and your surroundings. This makes you a different person from the one that started the book. I hope that by understanding the dangers of processed foods in causing weight gain and illness, and realizing the health benefits of natural foods, you will have noticed that your food preferences are changing. This identity change is the first and the most important step. You must feel the change from the inside first – when you act and think like a healthier person, your body catches up over the weeks and months that follow, taking on a new appearance. This feeling of a change in mindset should be empowering.

Habits play such an important role in how we go about our daily lives – they make up 45 per cent of our actions and are performed under the radar, without us being aware we made the decision to do them in the first place. The power that habits have on our lives is becoming more and more understood by researchers, but fortunately the science of habit change is advancing too. We can harness these scientific advances to help us change habits for the good, benefitting our health and quality of life.

The science of habit change tells us how to identify our bad habits and overwrite them with good ones. This is done by changing our environment, and by identifying and getting rid of the triggers that instigate the start of a bad habit and making the action to perform that habit more difficult. We can introduce other triggers that remind us to start a healthier habit and make that habit easy to perform. With repetition, those good habits will become an integral part of who we are. Something we perform automatically without the need for thought or willpower.

It's not just changing our eating habits that will affect our weight and health. Other aspects of our environment can alter our brain's weight anchor. These include:

- *Lowering our cortisol.* This stress hormone causes increased insulin and leads to weight gain (because the leptin signal is blocked). By trying to identify family and work stresses and dealing with them, we can reduce cortisol. Our body will respond by shifting that weight anchor back down.

- *Improving our sleeping pattern.* Melatonin is the sleepiness hormone that is released as dusk approaches. As the brain senses light decreasing, it readies the body for sleep by releasing this hormone. Unfortunately for many of us, this natural sleeping medicine is not released in time for bed. We live in homes and apartments that are well lit, and we stare at screens until late. No melatonin is released, and our sleep is disrupted. By dimming the lights an hour before bed and switching off our screens, we can reactivate our natural melatonin. The result is more restful sleep (7–9 hours minimum), which leads to a lowering of cortisol (see above) and makes de-stressing weight loss easier.

- *Exercise.* We have learned that extreme exercise is needed to push our weight down purely by calorie expenditure, so moderate exercise is not a cure-all for weight loss. We need an hour in the gym every day *plus* some sort of calorie restriction to override our metabolic adaptability – that ability to find savings in energy expenditure when needed. However, exercise is still great for us. It helps with insulin signalling and decreases cortisol. Exercise should be part of our daily routine – something we enjoy. Combined with healthy dietary changes and de-stressing, it will aid in weight loss.

De-stressing, a healthy sleeping routine and regular exercise are all important in helping our weight and health, but without dietary changes they will have little effect. The food we eat becomes us. The quality of our diet is the most important aspect for our future health. Make change easier by having that well-prepared kitchen space equipped with the correct utensils, a larder stocked with spices, herbs and other ingredients, and lots of fresh food in the fridge. Once you have planned your meals, it's then just up to you to hone your skills as a cook as you enjoy eating nutritious, healthy food.

In the final section of this book, there are some great meal ideas for you, your family and your friends to enjoy and savour.

Bon Appetit!

CHAPTER 12

Global Kitchen

'I was 32 when I started cooking; up until then I just ate.'

Julia Child

Lusaka, Zambia, September 1987

At the age of twenty-one I took a year off from medical school to work as a volunteer at a hospital in a remote part of Zambia in Africa. The year was eventful; there was a shortage of medical personnel so I was expected to act up as a doctor and midwife. I delivered many babies, crossed crocodile-infested waters to give emergency care, organized vaccination clinics, and even donated my blood to a bleeding patient before immediately assisting in the operation to stop the bleeding (while feeling very faint).

The day that I had arrived in Zambia I explored Lusaka, the bustling, humid capital city. In the evening, feeling very hungry, as I was trying to locate my hostel I saw a woman cooking on an open-air stove. She was frying onions, garlic, chillies and what looked like some sort of long, green vegetable. The aroma was mouth-watering. As is the case in most poor areas of the world, the people are the most generous, and sensing my hunger she plated up some of her food for me to try. It was wonderful – peppery, salty, with a touch of tangy flavour from the lime she squeezed onto it. The greens on the plate were nicely chewy and tasted of protein. I wanted to learn how to cook this; it was addictive and I'm sure very nutritious. 'What are these?' I asked, holding one of them, about to eat it . . .

She smiled. 'They are caterpillars, this is caterpillar season.'

The caterpillar season in Zambia is short. Sellers lay out a cloth on the floor and line up their hundreds of dried caterpillars for discerning buyers. I travelled the next day, so never had the opportunity to cook and savour pepper caterpillar again. I think that if I had known what was in the dish I would have baulked at it and never experienced its exotic taste. My culture and preconceived ideas of what to eat and what not to eat would have vetoed the idea of trying it.

Our Western cultural food norms can sometimes become a hindrance to changing our diets and the way we eat (and therefore who we are). For instance, many non-Western cultures don't have separate 'breakfast foods' like we do. They eat the same types of food in the morning as they would for the rest of the day. This tends to be much more nutritious and much less carbohydrate-heavy than our traditional Western breakfasts.

In the final chapter of this book I have laid out some recipe ideas for you to consider. These are designed to give you the nutrition that will help reduce the inflammation in your body and improve the function of your natural metabolic pathways. The recommended food in this lifelong programme will start to literally become the new you. You will no longer have a body that holds unnaturally high levels of omega-6, it will no longer be inflamed or bloated, and it will not want to hold on to fat stores and be sluggish. The tissues in your body will revert to a healthy ratio of inflammatory and anti-inflammatory omega fats, helping your insulin to work normally and freeing the weight-loss hormone leptin to be sensed by your brain. Natural weight loss will follow if this was your issue, or a natural settling of inflammation will follow if that was your concern. Avoiding huge amounts of sugar and unnaturally refined carbohydrates will also reduce your (now more efficient) insulin, unlocking leptin even more. Fructose will no longer signal for you to gain weight via those highly sweetened processed foods and carbonated drinks.

A note on the changes to your body. This change in the nutrition that you consume is not a quick fix. It can take up to twelve months of eating the correct foods for your body to change, as the omega fats take a while to move in and out. However, once your body metamorphoses to the new you, it is a lifelong fix. It really is that powerful. You will feel 100 per cent. Your body's metabolism will be fast, your immune system strong and your brain calm. You will become naturally slimmer, fitter and healthier . . . and because of this you will be more content with who you are.

I have laid out some guidance on breakfast (if required), lunch, dinner and snacks (also if required) in the following sections.

There are many natural healthy cuisines throughout the world – too many to cover in these pages – so I have tried to include a selection from different regions, including America, Africa, the Middle East, Europe and Asia. Each dish is specially selected not only to taste great and be easy to prepare but also to help optimal nutrition. Let these recipes become just the start of your food journey. More details of how to cook these recipes can be found at www.mymetabology.com. More dishes and eating ideas will appear on this website on a regular basis.

Metabology Nutrition*

- Reduce or cut out ultra-processed and fast foods from your diet.
- Use sugar and refined carbohydrates (such as wheat) as a cooking ingredient in moderation.
- Decrease the amount of omega-6 oil consumed, by cutting out vegetable oils† completely, and reducing the amount of natural foods high in omega-6 such as farm-fed chicken, beef and pork.
- Increase the amount of foods rich in omega-3 oils including wild (not farmed) fish, grass-fed beef, lamb and green leafy vegetables
- Do not avoid natural sources of saturated fat.
- Use salt freely in cooking.‡
- Try not to snack between meals if possible.
- Try using smaller plates.
- If possible, enjoy food with family and friends.
- If you cannot cook, try to learn how.

* *'Metabology' is a word introduced in my first book,* Why We Eat (Too Much). *It describes the study and understanding of our metabolism, what affects the flow of energy (calories) into and out of us, and our energy use and energy storage (in the form of fat).*

† *Sunflower oil, rapeseed oil, corn oil, cottonseed oil, canola oil, safflower oil, margarine, easy-spread fake butter, vegetable shortening.*

‡ *Salt can be used freely to add flavour to your cooking if you do not suffer with high blood pressure or related conditions. Please check with your doctor if you are unsure.*

Breakfast

Although some people say that breakfast helps you concentrate in the morning, there is no compelling reason that this meal is essential. Many people just don't feel that hungry in the morning. Our prehistoric ancestors would not have started eating as soon as they awoke. They would have gone out to hunt or gather food, driven by their hunger. Our bodies are not evolved to need food as soon as we rise.

We do know that eating only for a certain time period in the day is good for our insulin profiles and therefore our weight. In this respect, delaying eating in the morning is as good as stopping eating for the day in the early evening.*

If you tend not to be hungry in the morning, I would advise waking up your body with a drink of hot water mixed with the juice of a whole fresh lemon. This should start to get your metabolism firing in readiness for the day ahead. Although there are no scientific trials that prove that hot water and lemon in the morning is good for you (probably because the lemon industry never thought of sponsoring one), many people do this and many people find that it helps them. Things that stay popular tend to work, and I find this real-world evidence can be more powerful than many scientific trials.

If you are in a rush but want an easy nutritious breakfast, a great start to the day is fresh full-fat Greek yogurt sprinkled with berries and a little honey to taste. If you want a fast Arabic

---

* Time-restricted eating during the day for only eight or six hours, and for the rest of the time consuming zero-calorie drinks (water, herbal tea, black coffee), is a good habit to try to embrace.

breakfast, try black tea or coffee with three dates.* This should energize you just enough to start your day strongly.

The main foods to avoid for breakfast are the ones we often eat. Cereal, toast and orange juice (or any fresh fruit juice) will cause blood glucose fluctuations and therefore cravings for sugary foods throughout the rest of the day. Avoid these foods.

As mentioned, in many parts of the world the food consumed for breakfast can also be eaten at any time of the day. The Japanese, who are known for their health and longevity, often start their day with crispy fried or grilled salmon, some sticky rice, pickles, miso soup and green tea. In Trinidad and Tobago in the Caribbean, a commonly prepared breakfast is fry bodi, made from long green beans and tomatoes and accompanied by plantain or flatbread – a wonderfully tasty and high-protein start to the day. Costa Ricans eat gallo pinto in the morning, a delicious mix of rice and beans with sour cream, avocados and eggs. Try these for either breakfast or a meal later in the day.

TRADITIONAL JAPANESE BREAKFAST

Crispy Fried Salmon, Sticky Sushi Rice,
Miso Soup and Japanese Pickles

For the crispy fried or grilled salmon, pre-salt the *salmon* to taste. Leave the skin on and fry on this side until golden brown and crispy, then turn the salmon to cook through.

Place the *sushi rice* over the heat as soon as you have finished salting the fish, and cook to the instructions on the packet.

---

* Three dates to break a long fast is an Arabic tradition. It is said to be good for weight loss and libido.

Pre-prepared *miso soup* is acceptable, as fresh-made soup can be time-consuming.

For the Japanese pickles, finely slice (consider using a mandolin or potato peeler) *ginger/radish/cucumber/carrots* – mix with *white wine vinegar** and *salt* and *sugar* to taste.

Plate into separate small bowls, season with soy sauce and use chopsticks. Eat slowly and savour the food.

TRINIDADIAN BREAKFAST

Fry Bodi with Plantain or Home-made Flatbread

Fry 2 chopped ripe *plum tomatoes*, 1 *onion* and 7 crushed *garlic cloves* in a large sauté pan until soft. Add a bunch of long thin *green beans* and *salt* (2 tsp). Stir-fry over medium heat and cover for 10–15 minutes.

The bodi is ready when the beans begin to shrivel, turn colour, and any natural juices have evaporated or almost evaporated from them.

Serve hot or at room temperature with home-made *flatbread* or fried (or boiled) *plantain*. Remember hot pepper sauce to wake you up!

COSTA RICAN BREAKFAST

Gallo Pinto – Costa Rican Beans and Rice

Costa Rica has one of the healthiest populations in the world. They feature in the famous *Blue Zones* book which analyses areas of the world where people commonly remain healthy and active well into

---

* The acetic acid in the vinegar helps to lower the bloodsugar spike of the white rice.

their nineties. The traditional hearty Costa Rican breakfast is named *gallo pinto*, which literally means 'spotted rooster' – as the beans and rice resemble the speckling of a rooster's feathers.

Fry a chopped *onion* (white preferably) and a sweet *bell pepper* in olive oil for a few minutes until soft. Add 2 minced *garlic cloves* and simmer for a further minute. Add in 2 cups of *black beans* (with some of the liquid), 3 cups of *cooked rice* and ¼ cup of *salsa Lizano** (or Worcestershire sauce). Mix together well and cook for a further 3–4 minutes.

Plate up and sprinkle with chopped coriander. Gallo Pinto can be served with *yogurt, fresh tomato, sliced avocado* and *fried egg whites*. Pura vida!

Lunch on the Go

TIPS

- Bring food from home and store in a refrigerator at work.
- Cook extra food in the evenings and have for lunch the next day.
- Meal prep – batch-cook soups, stews, curries, roasted vegetables, chilli con carne, etc., to save time preparing meals in the week.
- Use a cool bag for salads, sandwiches, yogurt, etc., or a vacuum-insulated flask for soups and stews when on the go.

---

* Salsa Lizano is the national sauce of Costa Rica. It has sweet, spicy and earthy flavours. It's easily ordered online.

SALADS

How to build a salad:

1. **Choose a lean protein** such as grilled (grass-fed) beef or lamb, grilled salmon, prawns, tinned fish (in brine or tomato rather than oil), edamame beans, cottage cheese, feta, mozzarella, chickpeas or lentils.

2. **Add a selection of raw and/or cooked salad leaves and vegetables.** Try a range of textures and flavours including crunchy leaves (spinach, rocket, lettuce, shredded cabbage), sweet tomatoes, peppers, sweetcorn and grated carrot, hot radishes and chilli, savoury onions, creamy avocado, and cold cooked veg such as broccoli, green beans, asparagus and earthy roasted squash. You can even add fruit – try apple, pear, melon, peaches or grapes.

3. **Add a wholegrain or high-fibre carbohydrate** such as brown rice, quinoa (precooked sachets are fine), wholewheat pasta, couscous, new potatoes or roasted sweet potato.

4. **Add a healthy dressing.** Use extra-virgin olive oil with lemon or vinegar (keep separate, and shake and add just before eating), and add flavour with mustard, herbs, garlic, chilli, smoked paprika, soy sauce, miso or ginger. For a creamy dressing, use yogurt or avocado.

5. **Add interest with extras.** Add flavour and extra nutrients with a sprinkling of sesame seeds, capers, olives, pomegranate seeds, pickles or dried fruit.

HOT MEALS

Batch-cooking favourites – heat up at work, or bring in a vacuum-insulated flask.

- Home-made soups (lentil, vegetable, butternut squash)
- Stews and casseroles – use lean protein and plenty of veg
- Chilli con carne – use lean beef mince and bulk out with beans
- Ratatouille
- Vegetable frittata (using egg whites) or no-crust quiche
- Curries (spinach and chickpea, lentil dahl)

Snacks

TAKEAWAY SNACKS

- Rice cakes – these are a great go-to snack (top with avocado, soft cheese, tomato, etc.)
- Fresh fruit – fresh berries are best
- Chopped raw vegetables with a yogurt dip (add lemon, salt, sugar and fresh herbs to the yogurt to taste)
- Sliced lean meat – grass-fed beef or lamb
- Yogurt – choose high-protein Greek yogurt or Icelandic skyr where possible
- Edamame beans
- Comté cheese cut into squares
- Unsweetened (salted) home-made popcorn (not the microwave variety)
- Fresh fish pâté (see mackerel pâté recipe below)
- Tinned fish (in brine or tomato sauce, not in vegetable oil)

Mackerel Pâté

This is such a tasty and nutritious lunch, starter or snack. Buy ready-cooked *smoked mackerel* (around 250g/pack) and remove the skin. Add to your liquidizer with 120g *cream cheese*, a sprinkle of chopped *onions* (optional), 1 tsp *horseradish sauce*, the zest and juice of a *lemon* and some *parsley* or *coriander leaves*. Whisk into a pâté and transfer into small bowls.

Serve with home-made flatbread (see below) and chopped cucumber. Serves two.

Gluten-Free Flatbread

This gluten-free flatbread is the creation of my friend, the Cordon Bleu-trained, specialist gluten-free patisserie chef Fabiana. It has great texture, is tasty, and can be frozen if making a large batch.

Add ½ tsp *dry yeast* and 1 tsp *sugar* to 1.2 litres warm water (around 40 °C). Cover with foil until it dissolves (3 minutes). In a bowl, mix 150g *cassava flour*, 100g *rice flour*, 100g *oat flour*, 1 tsp *xanthan gum* and 1 tsp *salt*. Add 3 *egg whites* and 20ml *extra-virgin olive oil*.

Add the yeast water and knead into a dough and divide into 4–5 balls. Roll each into a thin circular patty and cook on a very hot skillet or non-stick frying pan (no oil needed) until browned on each side.

Pickles

Pickles are a great accompaniment to many dishes. They add an acidic, sour flavour that contrasts with and enhances other flavours in a dish. They can easily be home-made and can be ready to eat in an hour, and they keep in the fridge for up to two months. In Japan, it is normal to have a variety of home-made pickles available to choose from. Remember the fantastic metabolic effect of acetic acid in blunting sugar surges from carbohydrates.

Slice your choice of *mini cucumber/carrot/onion/cabbage/radish/ginger* (note that the denser or harder the vegetable, the finer the slicing needed, as the pickle will take longer to infuse) and add to sterilized recycled jars (plus *jalapenos* or *garlic cloves* to taste). Boil 2 parts *vinegar* (rice or wine vinegar is better) to 1 part water, ¼ part *sugar* and ⅛ part *salt*. Add *coriander seeds, mustard seeds* and *peppercorns*. Once boiled, remember to taste. If the mixture tastes good (sour, sweet and salty all in one), the pickle will be great. Pour into the jars and seal.

EVENING SNACKS

Raw Vegetable Charcuterie Board

Many people have a habit of snacking in the evening on poor-quality foods. My friend Samer's solution to this was not to give up this habit straight away but to replace the unhealthy snacks with healthy ones. Raw vegetables can be quite tasty, and they have minimal calories and contain great health-giving phytochemicals. A well-set-out vegetable charcuterie board should have nice colour combinations.

On a large wooden chopping board, arrange a selection of chopped raw vegetables, such as *cherry tomatoes, celery*, finely sliced (*red or white*) *cabbage, cucumber, carrots, sugar snap peas* or mini (or whole) sweet *bell pepper*. Dress with *salt* and *pepper* to taste, and consider serving with your own home-made ranch dressing.

For the dressing, mix full-fat *yogurt* (1 cup) with *Dijon mustard* (1 tsp), *buttermilk* (⅓ cup), and *chives, salt, pepper, onion powder, garlic powder* and *dried parsley* to taste. The ranch dressing can be poured into halved and hollowed-out bell peppers.

Meals

MIDDLE EAST

Lamb Koftas and Herbed Spelt

These Middle Eastern-inspired meatballs are flavoured with sumac, an earthy citrus-flavoured spice, and are oven-baked for ease and served over the super-grain spelt. Sprinkled with mint, spring onion and tomato, and served with thick Greek-style yogurt, there are hidden flavours all round with this dish.

Put oven on to high. Boil *spelt* (120g or half a mug) in a pot for 15–20 minutes. Chop up a handful of *dried cranberries* and a *garlic clove*. Mix this with half a pack (250g) of grass-fed *minced lamb* or *beef* plus *sumac* (1 tsp), *breadcrumbs* (30g), and *ground pepper* to taste. Divide into dumpling-sized balls (or sausage shapes) and bake in the oven for 12–15 minutes.

Dice a ripe *tomato* and finely chop a handful of *mint* and a little less of *spring onion*. Add these to the drained spelt and mix with a little *olive oil* and *salt* and *pepper*. This is the herbed spelt.

Mix up a splash of *olive oil* and *salt* and *pepper* with a third of a large pot of *yogurt*.

Serve the meat koftas over a bed of the herbed spelt and top with the yogurt.

LEBANON

Bulgur Pilaf

This is an easy and tasty recipe for bulgur wheat,* a healthy replacement for rice with higher protein, and lots of vitamins and minerals and health-giving phytochemicals. It is customizable, so the main ingredient of chickpeas can be swapped for peas, courgette, green beans, etc. Great as part of a main course accompanied by meat or fish, and served with salad and yogurt. Or it can be eaten on its own – just add a little olive oil, squeeze some lemon juice on top, and sprinkle with parsley leaves. Suitable the next day for a lunch on the go . . . or even breakfast.

Fry an *onion* gently in olive oil until starting to brown. Add 2 or 3 diced ripe *tomatoes*, a *green pepper* and *tomato paste*, and stir until the peppers soften and the tomato paste becomes aromatic (around 3–4 minutes).

Add 2 cups of *bulgur wheat*, fresh *cumin*, *salt* and *black pepper*, and mix until the bulgur is fully coated.

Stir in a cup of *chickpeas* (or sliced *green beans* or *courgette*).

Take the pot off the heat, add 3 cups of warm water (or stock), cover and leave for 10 minutes. Stir well to fluff up before garnishing.

Serving tip: overfill a small dome-shaped bowl with the pilaf, place your serving plate face down onto the bowl, and flip it all over so that the plate is now the right way up. Remove the bowl to leave a neat dome of pilaf (the same presentation can be used

---

* Bulgur wheat is parboiled whole cracked wheat. Because it uses the whole grain of wheat, none of the nutrients have been stripped away – it contains the germ, endosperm and bran. This makes it higher in protein, vitamins and minerals than regular white wheat flour, which contains only the endosperm and has minimal nutritional value.

to serve rice), which can be garnished with *parsley*, *lemon* and *olive oil*.

RUSSIA / ITALY

Mushroom Buckwheat Risotto

Buckwheat* is a heathy staple in Eastern Europe – especially Russia, where the population does not yet particularly suffer with obesity or an excess of Western-type diseases. This recipe is a fusion of the taste and health-giving benefits of buckwheat combined with the culinary tradition of an Italian risotto. Note that this recipe takes a lot less stirring and is quicker than a traditional Italian rice risotto.

Fry a finely diced *shallot* in 2 tbsp *olive oil* until soft. Add a cup of chopped *mushrooms* and cook until fully caramelized. Add a knob of *butter*, then pour in ½ cup coarse roasted *buckwheat* and stir until covered in oil. Add 1½ cups *vegetable stock* and bring to the boil. Add ⅓ cup grated *parmesan* and cook until reduced to a risotto consistency. Garnish with *parsley* or *chives*.

TURKEY

Coban Salatasi (Shepherd's Salad)

This typically Middle Eastern salad originates in Turkey but is popular in Greece and the Caucasus, particularly in the summer when its fresh ingredients are plentiful. Turkish shepherds would

---

* Despite its name, buckwheat has no relationship to wheat. It is a fruit seed from a plant related to rhubarb, and is therefore gluten-free. It contains high levels of protein, fibre and essential minerals. It has a pleasant subtle nutty flavour.

take tomatoes, cucumber and onions into the fields with them and make this salad to sustain them.

> Cucumber – peeled, deseeded and diced
> 3–4 tomatoes – diced
> Red bell pepper – diced
> 3–4 radishes – finely diced
> 2 spring onions – finely sliced
> Large bunch parsley – rolled tight and chopped
> 3 tsp *olive oil*, juice 1 *lemon*, 1 tsp *salt*, ½ tsp *pepper* – add to taste

MOROCCO

Moroccan Roasted Eggplant

Top and tail the *eggplant* (*aubergine*) and peel strips of skin lengthways to give a zebra pattern. Then cut across into 2.5cm (1-inch) pieces. Arrange the slices into rows on a baking tray lined with parchment paper, season with *salt* and *pepper* and drizzle with a coat of *olive oil*. Roast at high heat. Flip over halfway through, at 15 minutes.

In a bowl, mix finely chopped bunches of *parsley, coriander* and *dill*, some finely diced *dill pickles* (*gherkins*) and a *red pepper*, 2 cloves of finely sliced *garlic, salt* and *pepper* to taste, a pinch of *brown sugar, ground cumin, extra-virgin olive oil* and *white wine vinegar*. Leave for 15 minutes to marinate.

Place the roasted eggplant on a large platter and cover with the salad. Leave to cool for an hour in the fridge.

SOMALILAND

Lamb Maraq

Maraq is a delicious broth that is traditionally made in Somaliland and Yemen. It takes a while to cook the meat through, but actual preparation is short – everything goes into a pot and you just need to make sure that it doesn't dry out. It's extremely nutritious. Ask your butcher to dice the lamb on the bone.

Add diced *lamb shoulder* (on bone), chopped *onion* (1 or 2), *white cabbage, carrots, spring onions, green or red bell pepper,* 3 crushed *garlic cloves,* fresh spices (½ tsp each of *cumin, black pepper* and *turmeric,* some *cardamom pods* and *cloves,* a *bay leaf* and *salt* to taste)* and fresh *chillies* (optional) to a pot, and pour in water until the ingredients are covered.

Bring to a boil then turn down the heat. Regularly check that it's not drying out and spoon off the foam that collects on the surface. When the lamb is almost cooked (1–2 hours), add *potatoes* cut into large pieces and (1 tsp) freshly crushed coriander seeds. Cook for a further 30 minutes.

Leave to cool for 10 minutes before eating. Great on its own, or with flatbread or salad.

FRANCE

Fish with lemon beurre

A classic French fish dish with lemon sauce.

For the lemon beurre, sauté a finely sliced *shallot* and a thumb of *ginger.* As the onion is caramelizing, deglaze it with half a glass of *white wine.* Add *salt* and *pepper* to taste. Squeeze in the juice of half a *lemon.* Add a cup of *single cream.* In a cup, dissolve 1 tsp of *corn starch* in water. Add this to the sauce. Add cubes of *butter* until the

---

* Spices, apart from fresh ground coriander, are optional – add to taste. If they are not all available, don't worry.

sauce is a rich consistency. Blend in a liquidizer to bring out the shallot and ginger flavour.

Any type of *sea fish* can be used. Pre-salt the fish, then rub on a thin coat of *olive oil* and coat with a *flour* and *paprika* mix. Pan-fry the fish in butter with a small amount of olive oil, until cooked through. Serve with the lemon beurre sauce and garnish with *dill* and *lemon*.

INDIA

Paneer (or Meat) Jalfrezi with Cardamom Rice and Raita

Combining caramelized onion and green pepper in a rich tomato base, this version uses paneer cheese that's fried until golden and served with buttery cardamom rice and a yogurt raita. The paneer cheese has a healthy ratio of omega-3 to omega-6 fatty oils, so will have a great effect on your metabolism – even before the effect of the chillies! Grass-fed lamb or beef can be exchanged for the paneer.

For the jalfrezi, fry 200g of bite-sized cubes of *paneer* (or meat) in olive oil for 4–5 minutes until crispy golden brown. Transfer the paneer to a plate and fry a finely sliced *onion*, 1 tsp *salt* and 2 tsp *sugar* until caramelized. Add a sliced *green sweet pepper* and cook until softened. Add finely chopped fresh *ginger*, *garlic cloves* (2 or 3), *chilli pepper* (or ½ tsp chilli flakes) and 1 tbsp *curry powder*, and fry until the vegetables are coated. Add around 30–40g *tomato paste*, 2 sliced *tomatoes* and 300ml hot water mixed with a *vegetable stock cube*. Add the paneer, and cook until the sauce is reduced and the fresh tomato is soft.

Crush 6 *cardamom pods* (under a knife) and fry them in a saucepan with *olive oil* and a generous knob of *butter*. Add *basmati* rice (120g) and stir to coat the rice in the butter. Add 300ml cold water and bring to the boil. Once the surface of the boiling water reaches the top of the rice, turn the hob down low and cover. The rice needs no more attention and will be ready once the curry is cooked.

For the raita, mix together finely diced *cucumber*, a bunch of finely chopped fresh *coriander*, the juice of a *lemon*, full-fat *Greek yogurt*, *salt* and *sugar* to taste.

PERU

Rump Steak with Quinoa and Yogurt

Full of protein and fibre, this wholesome bowl is perfect after a busy day. The zingy chimichurri yogurt (packed with parsley, coriander, chilli, garlic and lemon) is delicious with the protein-rich steak, quinoa and fresh vegetables.

Boil 70g *quinoa* in water and reduce heat for 18–20 minutes until the water has absorbed into the quinoa.

Take 2 *rump, sirloin* or *fillet steaks* out of the fridge and pre-salt on both sides. Pat the steaks dry and coat them in *olive oil* and *cumin powder*. Fry the steaks in a very hot preheated frying pan (no need to add oil, as the steak is oiled) – 2 minutes on each side for medium rare, 3–4 minutes for medium to well done. Leave the steaks to rest on a chopping board. Slice a *red sweet pepper* into strips and fry until soft. Before serving, slice the steak into strips.

For the tomato salsa, mix (125g) quartered *cherry tomatoes* with a finely sliced *spring onion* and add ½ tbsp of *olive oil* and *salt* to taste.

For the chimichurri yogurt, finely slice a handful of fresh *coriander* and *parsley*, a *garlic clove* and a hot *red chilli pepper* (de-seeded), and crush into a paste with a pestle and mortar (add a small amount of water). Add the mixture to 80g full-fat *Greek yogurt* and fresh *lemon juice* and stir.

Remove the skin and stone and slice up an *avocado*.

Serve the steak slices, tomato salsa, yogurt and avocado on a bed of quinoa, and garnish with a wedge of *lemon*.

UNITED STATES OF AMERICA

New England Fish Chowder

The word 'chowder' originates from the French *chaudière* – a pot used to cook stews and soups in. This version of the dish is simple and adaptable. Vegetables can be switched depending on what you have available.

In a saucepan, fry a chopped *onion* and (2 or 3) *carrots* in *butter* until softened (small slices of *smoked bacon* can also be included to add a salty umami flavour). Add 3 large chopped *potatoes*, *sweetcorn* (frozen or tinned), a cup of *fish stock*, a *bay leaf*, and *salt, ground pepper* and *paprika* to taste. Add water to the pot until just covering the potatoes. Bring to the boil and simmer on a low heat for 15 minutes. Reduce the heat until the liquid is not simmering and add a cup of single cream (or milk). Stir until the chowder has thickened. Add 2 sliced *cod fillets* until cooked through, usually around 5 minutes (any white sea fish can be used, and clams and shellfish can also be added). Once cooked, stir in a bunch of finely chopped *parsley* and serve.

CHINA

Ho Fun Noodles

This tasty, filling and nutritious meal can be prepared in 15 minutes. Ho fun noodles are the flat, wide variety. Buy fresh rather than dried for a more authentic flavour.

In a wok, fry a chopped-up *onion* and a *sweet pepper* in *olive oil* for 3–4 minutes until softened. Add finely chopped fresh *ginger* and *garlic* to taste. Mix in *bok choy*. Push the vegetables to one side of the wok, and on the other side fry 3 *egg whites*. Once cooked, mix the egg whites with the vegetables. Add fresh wide *rice noodles*. Splash in some *sesame oil, rice vinegar, fish sauce, soy sauce* and a small amount of water. Stir-fry at high heat until the noodles are cooked.

Serve with a garnish of *sesame seeds* and *spring onion*.

For more information and recipe ideas, visit
www.mymetabology.com.

Acknowledgements

Following the success of my first book, *Why We Eat (Too Much)*, my publisher and my literary agent were relentless in trying to persuade me to write a follow-up. 'Don't leave it for too long,' they kept reminding me. But my problem was that I had no new ideas, and therefore no inspiration to write a sequel. This changed after my discussions with Samer Al Shraydeh, my Jordanian friend, on the psychological adjustment needed to sustain weight loss and health. Thank you, Samer, for your friendship and for the insights you gave me to inspire this second book.

Special thanks to Jamie Birkett, commissioning editor at Penguin Life, for his patient advice, and helping to guide the progress of the book as it unfolded. Gratitude in advance to my literary agent Elizabeth Sheinkman at PFD for her (future) work in helping the book reach a worldwide audience.

Appreciation to Angie Franklin (@therubicon) for guidance on medical communication and long-term strategy. Thanks to Malcolm Willett for his fantastic illustrations, which help to bring important concepts of the book alive.

I am indebted to Seema Yalamanchili, Muntzer Mughal, Abi Stevenson, Satish Chatwani, Bella James, Ella Hersi Farah and Alwyn Seeds for your conversations, enthusiasm and ideas for the book.

Cheers to the chefs! Henrietta Cottam, Audrey Johnson, Jennifer Lapish, Fabi Pragier (fabipragier.co.uk), Ria Birju (cookingwithria.com) and Gousto for their recipe contributions.

Thanks to my dietetic colleague Katherine Waller for her 'lunch on the go' suggestions.

To my colleagues at University College London Hospital: Maan Hasan, Wint Mon, James Holding, Andrea Pucci, Rachel Batterham, Marco Adamo, Mo Elkalaawy and Harry Markakis. Thanks, as ever, for your great teamwork and support.

Recognition to Eve Keighley and Dr Georgios Dimitriadis for their untiring work on *Obesity: The Big Truth*, which has helped the concepts of the weight set-point theory reach a wider audience of medical professionals.

In the UAE, thanks to my surgical colleague Dr Adriana Rotundo and her husband Flinn for their enthusiasm and encouragement, and to Dr Dina Elshamaa, consultant psychiatrist, for insights into how the mind works (and malfunctions). Appreciation to Prem Lobo and Aliah Poost for web and marketing help.

My office for literary, surgical and medicolegal work remains open, highly efficient and highly productive thanks only to my brilliant PA Natalie Cole. Thanks for keeping it this way even while I have been writing this book.

Finally, eternal gratitude to my family, who have as always been there to support me (and put up with me) with good humour and great food! Thank you for all your love.

Index

Page references in *italics* indicate images.

Index

fast food – *cont.*
restaurants 195–7
taste code and 64
unmasking 158–9
vegan 83
vegetable oils and 100, 199
See also processed foods; ultra-processed foods (UPFs)
fasting 7n, 183–4, 184n, 191
fat 3, 28, 34
burning 110
emulsifiers and 73
energy reserve and 34
essential 100–102
hibernation and 93–4
leptin and *see* leptin
omega 198, 199, 201
saturated 51, 66, 91n, 98, 99, 201, 202, 230
sleeve gastrectomy and 17, 18
sugar and 90–91
time-restricted eating and 191
weight loss and 7, 19–24, 20, 22
fenugreek 211
fermentation 49, 53, 55, 55n, 69
fibromyalgia 66, 81, 86, 200
fire, discovery of 53
fish
anti-inflammatory chemicals and 114, 201
brining 219
canned 207, 235, 236
Crispy Fried Salmon, Sticky Sushi Rice, Miso Soup and Japanese Pickles 232–3
Fish with Lemon Beurre 243–4
food pyramid and 67
frozen 209, 216
habit and 173
New England Fish Chowder 246
NOVA food classification system and 68

omega fats and 101, 201
pickles and 208
preserving techniques 55, 58
salt and 215, 220
ultra-processed foods and 69
wild 199, 201, 230
5′ nitrates (disodium 5′-ribonucleotides, E635) 61
flavouring, artificial 2, 31n, 47–8n, 66, 69, 76–9, 83, 114, 158–9, 221–2, 223
flavour enhancers 49
flavour industry 76
Food and Drug Administration (FDA), US 60, 76, 77
food delivery services 7, 83, 100, 148, 151, 157, 159, 173, 206, 216
food handicap horse race 157–8
food industry 3, 11, 48n, 65, 66, 70, 81, 82, 91n
advertising and 11, 154–9
eating habits and 152–9
food handicap horse race 157–8
priorities 152–3
food pleasure equation 63
food pyramid 67, 70
foods to avoid 197–200
foods to eat 200–202
frozen food 68, 69, 206, 208–9, 216, 237, 246
fructose
fruits and 201
high-fructose corn syrup (HFCS) 73n, 95–7, 100, 103–4
salt and 215
soft drinks and 52
sugar and 72n, 73n
weight set-point and 28, 44, 90, 92–7, 96, 100, 103–4, 111, 198, 199, 220
weight-gain switch 96–7, 96
Western diet and 31n, 44

256

Index